Human
SOLVING THE GLOBAL WORKFORCE
CRISIS IN HEALTHCARE

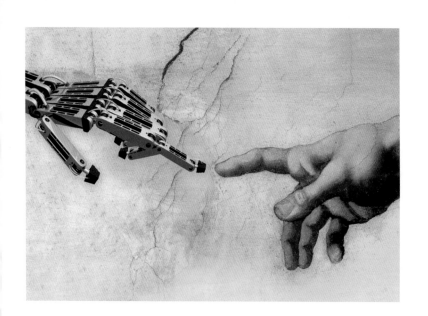

HUMAN
SOLVING THE GLOBAL WORKFORCE CRISIS IN HEALTHCARE

MARK BRITNELL

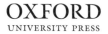
OXFORD
UNIVERSITY PRESS

Great Clarendon Street, Oxford, OX2 6DP,
United Kingdom

Oxford University Press is a department of the University of Oxford.
It furthers the University's objective of excellence in research, scholarship,
and education by publishing worldwide. Oxford is a registered trade mark of
Oxford University Press in the UK and in certain other countries

First Edition published in 2019

Impression: 1

Published in the United States of America by Oxford University Press
198 Madison Avenue, New York, NY 10016, United States of America

British Library Cataloguing in Publication Data

Data available

Library of Congress Control Number: 2018962717

ISBN 978–0–19–883652–0

Printed in Great Britain by
Bell & Bain Ltd., Glasgow

In memory of my mother, Veronica
For my children, Reuben and Beatrix Britnell

Foreword by Nigel Crisp

This is a timely and optimistic book which should be a guide to politicians and practitioners alike.

There is a great deal of wisdom in these pages and it contains many eminently quotable phrases, examples, and figures; but perhaps the book's greatest achievement is to rebalance the whole health debate. It moves us away from a purely economic and technological approach to focus on the human.

Health and healthcare are ultimately about people, relationships, communities, trust, what we value, and how we want to live our lives. Health is, in philosopher Amartya Sen's words, a core part of 'human flourishing'. Mark Britnell reminds us of this at every step of the way.

He draws out many important themes. Health workers could do even more than they do now if they were enabled to work to the top of their licence. Nurses—half the professional health workforce—are perhaps the prime example, with many reporting that they can't work at the level they are trained to do, an extraordinary waste of talent and resources. We are just beginning to see the development of new and innovative nurse-led and nurse-based services as part of the wider development of new models of care.

Innovation comes from all parts of the world, as Britnell demonstrates. People in low- and middle-income countries can be great innovators. Without the baggage of history, they can *Turn the World Upside Down* as I have written elsewhere. We can all learn from them about, for example, the involvement of communities, carers, and relatives as partners with the professionals.

It is, as Britnell argues, human beings who will make improvement happen—aided by the wonders of technology and supported by the better use of resources. As a result, he argues persuasively that we should 'entirely reframe and reposition the debate about workforce planning to one of productivity, health, and national wealth creation'.

Mark Britnell brings to his writing all the experience he has gathered from working in countries all around the world. He has been a successful health service leader and policymaker in his own country and has since gained the broadest possible overview of health globally through running a flourishing worldwide enterprise. His passion, knowledge, and enthusiasm are evident on every page. He is ideally placed to guide us all in improving health through emphasizing the human.

Lord Nigel Crisp, Co-Chair of the All-Party Parliamentary
Group on Global Health and of Nursing Now,
formerly Chief Executive of the NHS

Preface: Cognitive dissonance

'The greatest danger for most of us is not that our aim is too high and we miss it, but that it is too low and we reach it.'
Michelangelo 1475–1564

The truism that 'there is no healthcare without the workforce' is universally acknowledged but poorly acted upon. We are hurtling towards a global workforce crisis in healthcare because of a growing and ageing population which places greater needs and demands on health at just the time when the ratio of employed workers to older people and other dependents has never been more challenging, while the millennial generation is far less inhibited about changing jobs and careers. Put simply, in healthcare, we face a future where there is too much work with too few workers.

Yet across the globe there are politicians and health employers who manage to exhibit amazing levels of cognitive dissonance; they seem able to hold contradictory ideas and values simultaneously. They proclaim their love for healthcare staff yet persistently underappreciate them; they celebrate the extra jobs created but fail to plan for a healthy supply of staff to fill them; and they extol the benefits of technology without planning for enormous digital disruption. In short, they say one thing and do another.

We have reviewed hundreds of papers and articles worldwide on the healthcare workforce for this book. With notable exceptions, they concentrate on immediate and imminent staffing problems and fall short of serious, joined-up strategic solutions. Many are written from a laudable but narrow professional view. There is little real coordination between the clinical practitioners, educationalists, researchers, scientists, technologists, demographers, economists, workforce specialists, and health executives, let alone patients and the public. But as humans we can decide to solve this problem if we want to, and work more collaboratively and imaginatively. We have to raise our ambitions.

The cover of the book is immediately recognizable. *The Creation of Adam* is a fresco painted by Michelangelo between 1508 and 1512 in the Sistine Chapel in Rome. It was inspired by the Book of Genesis, and the picture of the outstretched hands of God and Adam has become the iconic image of humanity. The book cover replaces the hand of Adam with that of a robot, forged through technology. I chose the image because I firmly believe that humankind is capable of solving the global workforce crisis with the help of the technology it has created. But technology should always be subordinated to human needs, and forms but one part of the solution. The book is called 'Human' because the essence of healthcare is compassion, empathy, and humility, offered with dignity and respect. These enduring human attributes will not be replaced by machines because, at the greatest times of illness and vulnerability, the kind heart and warm touch of a human can lift the spirit.

This book is written with a timeframe of 10 years or so in mind, to 2030. In 2017 the Fourth Global Forum on Human Resources for Health, convened in the Irish capital by the World Health Organization and others, described in stark terms the crisis facing us. The Dublin Declaration on Human Resources for Health said we will need around 40 million more healthcare workers by 2030, but we are in danger of being 18 million short[1]—more than one in five of the 80 million[2] we will need. It called for countries across the globe to increase health financing and the recruitment, development, training, and retention of healthcare workers.

The chapters that follow do not—indeed cannot—offer quick fixes, but show how this gap could be closed through orchestrated policy and action across a number of fronts. My ideas are based on what I have seen working with both humans and technology during my global travels. If all these approaches were pursued, the total number of healthcare staff needed would be considerably fewer than the current target—but still many more than we have today.

I am not a futurologist, digital wizard, or workforce specialist but have, over the past 10 years, worked around the world in 77 countries on about 330 occasions helping to improve healthcare. Over my 30-year career dedicated to health services I have had the privilege of leading organizations at local, regional, national, and global levels, payer and provider, public and private sectors, and passionately believe in the extraordinary abilities of staff. For example, during my time at University Hospital Birmingham (UHB), one of the largest employers in the NHS, 86% of staff said they were 'proud to work for UHB'. I am now Global Chairman and Senior Partner for Healthcare, Government, and Infrastructure at KPMG International. KPMG can trace its roots back more than 150 years, and is now a worldwide network of professional services firms spanning 157 countries. It is consistently ranked in or around the top 10 employers worldwide. I hope my experience and observations help practitioners and policymakers alike solve the workforce challenge that we face together over the coming decade.

The chapters that cover various countries across the continents are designed to give a flavour of their workforce issues rather than provide a compilation of all the details. I have tried to juxtapose the chapters on themes, such as technology or the role of government, with countries that highlight some of the issues raised.

I want to acknowledge that this book does not talk sufficiently about all health professions. It is axiomatic that allied health professionals, clinical scientists and a whole range of other dedicated staff make healthcare what it is today but, unfortunately, we just couldn't find enough consistent data across countries with which to work. Sadly, this is also true for social care and human services, both vital partners in health and well-being.

I have tried to be even-handed with the facts, but these inevitably change as the world turns and health systems move on. That said, unfortunately, developments in healthcare workforce are often glacial in nature. This short book is not designed to be an academic compendium and, as we all have busy lives, each chapter can be read in the time it takes to drink a cup of coffee.

Written in a personal capacity on planes, trains, and automobiles, this book could only have been completed with the research, drafting, and editing skills of Dr Charlotte Refsum, Dr Edward Fitzgerald, Jonty Roland, and Richard Vize. They have been magnificent and it has been great fun working as a team.

I would also like to thank the clients, colleagues, and countries I have worked with and in. I am privileged to work globally and it has given me a deep appreciation of how diversity and cultural difference can spur creativity, innovation, and goodwill to new heights. My gratitude is also extended to the 16-strong International Review Panel who are acknowledged along with others at the end of the book.

As I said in my first book, *In Search of the Perfect Health System*, we all have something to teach and something to learn. The Roman statesman and philosopher Seneca once said, 'travel and change of place impart new vigour to the mind'. I certainly believe this to be true, and hope you enjoy the book.

Mark Britnell
Spring 2019
London

Contents

Chapter 1

Introduction: A workforce solution is within our grasp

Over the past decade while working all over the world, I have come to the regrettable conclusion that no country—rich or poor—manages its health workforce and workforce needs particularly well. Many countries are awash with analysis which painstakingly outlines looming shortages and crises, but there are few examples of excellent practice which improves the situation for the long term. Countries and organizations often try to spend their way out of problems with short-term fixes, causing more problems for others and, ultimately, themselves.

This is a big global problem now and it will worsen over the next decade. Since the beginning of this century the health and social care workforce has grown rapidly, but it is still not enough. Projections indicate that by 2030 demand for health workers will rise to 80 million,[1] but the World Health Organization estimates there will be a worldwide shortage of around 18 million, more than one in five of the people we will need.[2]

I have three motivations for writing this book. First, as I have been travelling I have noticed how my conversations with health leaders have changed. Immediately after the global financial crisis of 2008 most health systems were obviously obsessed with money (usually the lack of it). While this has not disappeared, it is increasingly overshadowed by the realization that we simply do not have enough staff to care for patients. Second, I do not believe we have to sleepwalk into this problem. With concerted, coherent effort we can supply sufficient healthcare staff, reimagine service delivery, harness technology, extend healthy life expectancy, and increase the economic well-being of nations by 2030. Health is wealth. Finally, I believe that by orchestrating 10 large-scale changes—affecting everything from how we make our staff feel loved, to how we manage the interaction of humans and robots—we can increase the capacity to care by roughly 20%—thus meeting the anticipated shortfall in staff. Box 1.1 illustrates the themes that are discussed in greater detail in the chapters that follow, while the country chapters highlight what their health systems can teach others, along with the challenges they face.

My central argument, therefore, is that we are facing a workforce crisis which is a 'wicked problem' needing a lot more than the usual linear management solutions. The complex adaptive challenge requires us to think, work, and collaborate in different ways. No country or health system is yet consistently addressing the 10 priorities for change I have identified. We need to reframe the productivity debate, reimagine clinical services, and change national investment strategies, as well as harnessing the disruptive power of technology and artificial intelligence (AI).

Staff shortages will not be spread evenly over health systems but they will be experienced everywhere. Growth in the demand for health workers will be highest

Box 1.1 Ten large-scale changes to tackle the global health workforce crisis

1 Reframe and reposition the debate about workforce planning to one about productivity, health, and national wealth creation.

2 Encourage governments to become more entrepreneurial, stimulating health worker supply through a host of measures ranging from the relaxation of training limits to increased labour participation rates for healthcare.

3 Encourage the rapid and large-scale adoption of new models of care that already exist in different parts of the world so that enhanced well-being, prevention, promotion, care, and treatment can increase productivity and capacity to care.

4 Provide the human and technological support to enable patients to be active partners in their care, taking greater responsibility for their own well-being and the management of long-term conditions. This should be a given in the twenty-first century.

5 Provide greater recognition, encouragement, and support for communities, volunteers, and families, who already provide most of the care in society.

6 Support health professionals to practise at the upper limits of their clinical licence, encouraged by regulators.

7 Create a new cadre of peripatetic care assistants and workers who seamlessly straddle health and social care to deliver services in communities, hospitals, and homes.

8 Stimulate the disruptive digital possibilities offered by AI, cognitive assistance, robotics, and blockchain to increase time to care and productivity; healthcare has little to fear and much to gain from the rise of the intelligent machine.

9 Instead of passively waiting to be shaped by the impact of digital technology and machines on the workforce, organizations need to become agile, learning systems which educate, re-educate, and support workers, to gain productive and competitive advantage and maximize staff well-being.

10 The healthcare industry needs to overhaul its rudimentary approaches to the leadership, development, and coaching of individuals and teams, embracing proven techniques which raise motivation and performance.

among upper-middle-income countries, driven by growing economies, populations, and ageing. These shortages will fuel global competition for skilled health workers at just the time that nationalism and nation-first politics are gaining popular traction. Middle-income countries will face shortages as demand exceeds supply, and low-income countries will face low growth in both demand and supply and will not be able to meet the United Nations' Sustainable Development Goals for health and well-being, which set ambitious targets for disease reduction and health equity including universal health coverage by 2030. Every country signed up to the Development Goals, but they now need to spell out how they will play their part in delivering universal health coverage, ensuring they make their fair contribution to the pool of global health talent. These are life and death issues.

Universal health coverage is a just cause, given that the average life expectancy of a citizen born in Sierra Leone is just 50 years compared with the 84 years lived in Japan[3]—a terrible waste of life and human potential. Of course, this is not just a problem for developing countries. A man born in upmarket Kensington, London, can expect to live for 83 years while a man born in Glasgow, Scotland, would be expected to live just 73 years. In America, Oglala Lakota County, South Dakota—which includes the Pine Ridge Native American reservation—has the lowest life expectancy at 66 years, while a cluster of counties in Colorado enjoy 86 years of life.[4]

The greatest gift a country can give its people

Universal healthcare is the greatest gift any country can give its people, but we are currently on a trajectory of failure condoned by those who passively accept that demography is destiny. All too often I have found some health professionals and academics have been more eager to analyse the problem than mobilize for action.

Unfortunately, many health systems fail to put their best people on the most important problem—the future supply, management, and motivation of healthcare staff. In some respects, it is a Cinderella service. Many health organizations and systems are still stuck in the mindset of thinking about personnel issues. Instead, we need a fundamental reset of approach to ensure a relentless focus on human resources. Hospital and health system governing boards should—at the very least—give 'people' the same priority as 'finance'.

No one country has all the solutions, but I am convinced we can generate the equivalent of 20% extra capacity to care over the next decade or so if politicians, policymakers, practitioners, patients, and the public change their ways. Of course, it is difficult, but it is an urgent priority if we are to provide adequate healthcare for all 8.5 billion humans that will live on the planet by 2030. This is an honourable goal which is attainable if we leverage the best ideas around the world, orchestrate effort nationally, and learn from other sectors of the economy that have changed more rapidly to harness the technological power of the fourth industrial revolution.

Fractured globalization

All over the world people ignore the blessings associated with globalization while being quick to point to its failures. Over the past 25 years, globalization, liberal democracy, and free-market economics have faced a crisis of identity in the West and parts of the East. People are troubled and find it hard to know what their country stands for now. Growing numbers of middle-class citizens feel they have neither adequate security nor liberty. The poor have always felt this. The young and the old feel alienated in different ways. Many feel their country is moving away from them—caring less for them as their standard of life stalls or falls. When people feel their opportunities are diminished they look for quick and simple answers, which is when populism takes hold.

Decent healthcare can help heal these fractures. Health is cited as a top five political issue for most countries. Governments are a little bit similar to Maslow's 'hierarchy of needs'. As a first base, functioning societies and democracies need to provide security for their populations—military security, economic security, social security, and health security. Only when these are in place do liberty and the legitimacy of democratic institutions flourish.

Health has an enormous role to play in building hope and social cohesion, and a well-trained, technologically productive health workforce is good for families and society and their economies. The enduring values of healthcare—compassion, fairness, and equity—can bring people together. But there is a problem.

Currently standing at just over $9 trillion, the global healthcare sector is the second largest industry in the world, consuming an average of around 10% of a country's gross domestic product (GDP). Yet the capability and capacity for the industry to replenish itself, innovate, and become more productive is frustratingly slow and amateur. Coupled with the workforce shortages, this slothfulness will cause unnecessary deaths, impede the healthy extension of life, and slow the growth of national wealth and harmonious societies. It doesn't have to be this way.

An enormous challenge

The health sector globally is performing poorly on predicting and delivering numbers of properly trained health workers. The World Health Organization and Global Health Workforce Alliance looked at workforce data for 183 countries covering supply, skills, access to care, and the dignity of care and concluded that every single one of them had staff shortages.[5]

The workforce is ageing and not being sufficiently replaced. Availability and accessibility are highly uneven in their spread (there are substantial issues of geographical equity for health professionals within countries, let alone between them). Health worker motivation is problematic in many countries and performance assessment and management of individuals is rudimentary and given insufficient priority. Countries' capacity to estimate future human resource needs and design longer term policies is highly variable. Quality information and reliable data is problematic. There is a pressing need to rethink how staff are trained, deployed, and rewarded.

Lying behind these difficulties are hard numbers and human lives. The *British Medical Journal* reports that China is short of at least 200,000 paediatricians, 161,000 general practitioners, and 40,000 psychiatrists.[6] A high-ranking health official in Beijing told me that the relaxation of the 'one child' policy (to maintain economic growth and support an ageing population) would require an extra 180,000 obstetricians by 2022. It has been estimated that India requires an extra 1.5 million doctors and 2.4 million nurses just to match the global average, while the physicians that do exist live in the cities, which only account for a third of India's mainly rural population.[7] While working in India recently, hospital officials confided to me that the government's desire to double the amount of public health expenditure to 2.5% of GDP might fail because the human capital simply does not exist, so the extra money would push up wages rather than deliver sustainable jobs growth.

In Japan the number of nurses tripled from 550,000 in 2000 to 1.7 million in 2013 yet incredibly, according to the *Japan Times*, the country is now seeking to add an extra 250,000 nurses from 2017. According to the Ministry of Welfare, Japan will also need 2.5 million care workers by 2025 but estimates it will fall short by 377,000 because its population is ageing and declining as the fertility rate decreases. Germany expects to be 300,000 nurses short by 2030.[8]

In the United States, according to the Bureau of Labor Statistics, 1.2 million vacancies will emerge for registered nurses between 2014 and 2022.[9] This is being driven by the ageing of the Baby Boomer generation, with the percentage of people aged over 65 forecast to rise by 75% to 69 million, meaning one in five Americans will be a senior citizen.[10] In a double whammy, around one million registered nurses are older than 50, suggesting that nearly one-third of the current workforce will retire in the next decade.[11] To add insult to injury, a recent survey of chief nursing officers revealed that 61% thought nurse shortages were harming nurse morale and more than a third said it was having a considerable impact on patient care.[12]

For doctors, a report by the Association of American Medical Colleges reveals that the physician shortage is getting worse as the population grows and ages. By 2030 the shortfall is expected to total anywhere between 41,000 and 105,000[13] (a perfect example of unreliable data) depending on numerous factors including immigration policies. Yet it would be foolish to write America off. During the Obama years, in a push to become the final Organisation for Economic Co-operation and Development (OECD) member to provide universal healthcare, his reforms contributed to total growth in healthcare staff of more than 1.5 million staff. That is phenomenal, adding roughly the equivalent of the entire workforce of the United Kingdom's National Health Service (NHS)—itself the fifth largest employer in the world[14]—in just five years. If one considers that only 40% of the world's countries currently have universal healthcare, it is not difficult to imagine the global 'war for talent' that has been ignited by the Sustainable Development Goals, which have resulted in countries across the globe committing to universal health coverage by 2030.

In the United Kingdom, Brexit could have profound consequences for the health workforce and patient care. The near total collapse in European Union (EU) nurses registering to work in the United Kingdom (worsened by the introduction of a tougher language test for migrant nurses) has aggravated an already chronic problem. While the number of NHS clinicians has risen by 26,000 since 2012, this has been outstripped by the creation of 62,000 additional posts, including many established in the wake of the Mid Staffordshire hospital crisis, where insufficient nursing staff was associated with a higher than expected number of patient deaths.[15] In June 2018 there were almost 42,000 unfilled nursing posts in the NHS in addition to 62,000 staff, or 5.6% of all NHS workers, classified as EU nationals. Overall, 12% of NHS staff say their nationality is not British.[16] So even where countries and health systems can afford to create extra clinical posts, the staff increasingly do not exist.

While my travels have taken me to many interesting places, there are more which I have yet to explore fully. For example, the Middle East and the Gulf Cooperation Council (GCC), representing six countries including Saudi Arabia and the United Arab Emirates (UAE), all have particular workforce challenges alongside ambitious strategies for healthcare sustainability. I have visited Saudi Arabia, Qatar, and the UAE and marvelled at their ability to establish impressive healthcare infrastructure. But despite good salaries and low taxation rates the workforce challenges are a persistent problem, including the reliance on staff from abroad.

In Saudi Arabia and the UAE, the proportions of expatriate healthcare workers are 78% and 85%, respectively. The GCC has 5.5 nurses per 1,000 population, compared with the United States at 11.3 and Germany at 13.3. Only 3% of the nurses in the UAE are Emirati.[17] Competition for skilled healthcare workers among the GCC is fierce and bound to increase. So even with massive financial resources, countries cannot entirely buy their way out of workforce shortages.

The global movement of clinical skills is insatiable, and as Figure 1.1 shows, medical migration in full flow. More countries are opening doors to foreign-trained physicians, with Israel topping the league with 58% of all its doctors trained abroad. This is followed by Australia at 30%, the United Kingdom at 28%, United States at 25%, and Canada at 23%.[18]

Of course, it is not just doctors who move around the world. Chris Tufton, the health minister of Jamaica, explained to me that the loss of nursing personnel across the Caribbean is creating a crisis in the delivery of health services in vulnerable countries such as his. He cites a World Bank report of 2009 which revealed that, 15 years after graduation, about half the nurses from English-speaking Caribbean countries were working abroad. He estimated that the regional shortage of nurses was expected to triple to over 10,000 by 2030, just as many countries across the Caribbean are launching national health insurance and universal healthcare schemes. More dramatically, in Africa, 25% of the world's disease burden confronts just 4% of the healthcare workforce.

How did we get into this mess?

Some countries can afford more healthcare workers and can find them, some can afford more workers but cannot find them, some produce more workers than they can afford, and some can neither afford nor find health workers. Some countries believe in free market forces to shape labour supply while others take a more state regulated and planned approach to future workforce needs. Most health systems can point to small-scale, local success but many countries can see that whatever efforts they make are overwhelmed by the magnitude of the demographic, labour, and service delivery challenge. It's all been too little, too late.

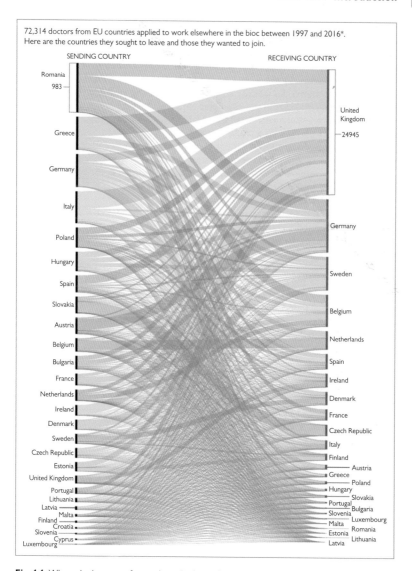

72,314 doctors from EU countries applied to work elsewhere in the bloc between 1997 and 2016*.
Here are the countries they sought to leave and those they wanted to join.

Fig. 1.1 Where do they come from, where do they go?

Reproduced with permission from Hervey, G/POLITICO. The EU exodus: When doctors and nurses follow the money. POLITICO. 9/27/17. Copyright © 2017 POLTICO. Available at https://www.politico.eu/article/doctors-nurses-migration-health-care-crisis-workers-follow-the-money-european-commission-data/

According to Deloitte, doctors and nurses are more likely to move between countries than people in any other highly regulated profession, driven by better pay and opportunities.[19] The pattern of migration it identifies in Europe has wider resonance. Within the continent, professionals tend to move from east to west and south to north—in other words, towards the better resourced and better paying health systems. So poorer countries are training staff for their wealthier neighbours. It is striking that the countries with the highest proportion of foreign-trained nurses are Switzerland (19%), the United Kingdom (15%), and Norway (9%).[20]

But the drivers of migration are more complex than just pay and resources. They include historical, political, and trade relationships, workforce policies, supply and demand, demographic trends such as the number of women in the workforce, and migrant licensing and registration rules, much of which may have nothing to do with the needs of the local healthcare system.[21]

Policy changes can drive sharp shifts in immigration. In the United Kingdom, for example, the number of migrant doctors and nurses rose rapidly in the early 2000s, before dropping sharply from 2006 to 2008 as the government ended its international recruitment drive.[22]

The World Health Organization (WHO)'s study of healthcare migration patterns in the aftermath of the global financial crisis highlights the complexity of supply and demand. India was the top country of origin for doctors in Australia, the United Kingdom, and the United States. South Africa has been a major supplier to Australia, the United Kingdom, and Canada, while the United States was the largest origin country for Canada.[23]

The Philippines was the dominant country of origin for nurses, being the top source for Canada, the United Kingdom, and the United States. In Australia, the top three sources for nurses were New Zealand, the United Kingdom/Ireland, and the Philippines. The United States attracts substantial numbers from Mexico and Haiti, and the United Kingdom still attracts considerable numbers from former colonies.

Pay differentials can be massive. A Filipino nurse might earn 20 times more in the United States than at home. Remittances—money sent home to the family—are an example of the conflicting impact of migration. Huge numbers of staff sending money back is good for the economy but makes it difficult for the Philippines' healthcare system to keep good staff.

Professional regulation can be a significant barrier to migration, with wide variation in the rules governing the registration of nurses, midwives, and doctors. Registration systems are often poorly adapted to registering migrants, and the reason for arriving in a country—such as joining one's family or claiming political asylum—can be another barrier. Perceptions matter too. I have come across plenty of examples of doctors quitting the United Kingdom for Australia because they expect the work to be less pressurized and bureaucratic.

The impact on developing countries

A major study by Nair and Webster (2012) into the impact of health professionals' migration on developing countries identified three distinct flows—one between countries and two within them. Internationally, staff tend to migrate from south to north, while within developing countries they tend to move from rural to urban areas and from public sector to private or non-governmental organizations (NGOs).[24]

Nair and Webster found significant shifts from public to private in countries such as India, Thailand, and China. The growth in medical tourism is leading to an upsurge of private and multinational hospitals which often hire the best specialists, to the detriment of the public healthcare system. NGOs can exacerbate problems by hiring the best staff on good pay.

Supply and demand can have some unexpected effects. In the Philippines, doctors have been retraining as nurses because of the higher international demand, while in China, doctors struggling to compete with a growing market for overseas physicians are moving into research and jobs with pharmaceutical companies.[25]

The Migration Policy Institute examined the impact of healthcare workers' migration on Malawi.[26] The first medical school opened in 1991. A decade later more than half of the 500 doctors born and trained in Malawi were working abroad, as were around one in six of the 2,200 home-trained nurses. Popular destinations included the United States, South Africa, and the former colonial power of the United Kingdom.[27]

Emigration led to chronic staff shortages. By 2004 there were 250 doctors for a population of 23 million, and half the doctors worked in the cities even though the population was overwhelmingly rural. The Ministry of Health described the health sector as 'critical, dangerously close to collapse . . . facing a major, persistent and deepening crisis with respect to human resources'.

It launched a six-year Emergency Human Resources Programme to raise staffing levels. The $100m investment over five years attracted major donor funding, notably from the United Kingdom's Department for International Development. The major groups of staff were given pay increases of around 50%, the numbers being trained were increased and volunteers were brought in to plug short-term gaps. Incentives encouraged staff to work in rural areas, the availability of drugs and medical supplies was improved, and poor management was tackled.

By the end of the programme the number of healthcare workers per 100,000 population had increased by about two-thirds and there has been a sharp decline in migration. But the workforce is still significantly smaller than the African average.

It is important to bear in mind that, as the report Triple Impact from the United Kingdom's All-Party Parliamentary Group on Global Health highlighted, migration is only one part of the workforce problem confronting low- and middle-income countries. It states: 'For example, it has been estimated that if every African health worker who had received some level of health worker training and then emigrated were to return home, this would only address about 10% of the shortage in the continent. There are many interconnected problems but in numbers terms the single biggest factor is that not enough nurses and other health workers are trained in the first place.'

Nonetheless, healthcare migration is still a big issue. In 2010 the obvious problems it was causing prompted the 193 member states of the WHO to adopt the Global Code of Practice on the International Recruitment of Health Personnel.[28] It describes the responsibilities of everyone from governments and recruitment agencies to the staff themselves, trying to balance the obligations of healthcare workers to the country in which they were trained with their right to find work abroad.

It committed countries to promote the sustainability of healthcare systems in developing countries, and to improve their own health workforce planning, education, training, and retention to reduce the need to attract migrant staff.

While the global commitment to the code of practice is a promising step, it is difficult to discern a significant impact. Analysis of its first few years indicates that progress is patchy at best.[29] To truly meet the size of the challenge, global action needs to be sustained, radical, and imaginative.

Short-term thinking

All over the world, I have seen how health systems and organizations repeatedly tackle the urgent rather than important issues. It is easy to see why. Faced with ever-increasing patient demand as populations age, grow, and carry a greater burden of non-communicable disease, health systems have to deal with immediate pressures. Some take the workforce for granted and nearly all health systems have been blithely assuming that someone will always be there to cope with the work. Workforce planning is technically difficult because the periods over which forecasts are made are long and the impacts of new models of care are difficult to compute.

At least some of the workforce planning failures are the result of unrealistic expectations from politicians and policymakers disconnected from delivery. Workforce planning is often isolated from clinical and financial planning. A high proportion of education and training costs are spent upfront on attracting new recruits—driven by competing professional silos and interest groups—while fewer resources are committed to developing the existing workforce and ensuring the right skills exist in the right numbers in the right place at the right time. Workforce planning requires the ability to respond flexibly to different supply and demand factors over time. As the King's Fund has pointed out, it is less about long-term predictive precision than about developing an adaptive, flexible approach.

Solving the problem—by 20%

Surely it can't be that difficult? After all, we managed to sequence the human genome back in 2003 after more than a decade of endeavour, and that was a rather harder challenge. But while other industries take much more flexible, agile approaches to managing their workforce needs, human resource management in healthcare is much more about process than practice. I am not a workforce or human resource specialist, but I am convinced this problem can be solved. Over the following chapters I outline a series of actions that, when taken together, can improve workforce capability and the capacity to care by 20% or so.

Leading—not resisting—the productivity debate

The debate in healthcare about workforce supply, sufficiency, and pay has taken place on the wrong territory. For the next decade, the discussion needs to address productivity head-on. Across the world, productivity in healthcare has been lack-lustre. I used to think that care process redesign and quality improvement techniques such as Lean could modernize care pathways and improve productivity. While this is sometimes true, I have increasingly come to recognize that many of these worthy initiatives, which often take years, fail because managers realize too late that they have not got the clinical skills they need in the right place at the right time, and in the right quantity and quality.

If we are to have sufficient healthcare staff enhancing population health and national wealth, then management and investment strategies for staff and technology need to be radically different. While it is easy to highlight the difficulty of assessing the true productivity of healthcare, given the numerous ways we can judge and measure patient outcomes, it is now essential we do so.

Like other industries, productivity usually grows through four major sources: improving the well-being and health of the workforce (reducing absenteeism); investing in training, education, and development (skills); introducing new forms of technology (efficiency); and innovating with new care and business models (effectiveness). In America healthcare productivity has actually decreased by 0.6% annually over the past 20 years compared with 2.5% growth across the entire economy, while in the United Kingdom, NHS productivity grew at 0.8% per year from 1995 to 2015[30] (about half the rate of the entire economy). If health is to generate greater national wealth then it is vital to link the health and well-being of the workforce explicitly with productivity, so governments and business make the necessary long-term investment to realize this ambition.

For example, Australia has enjoyed its longest period of economic prosperity, yet its productivity growth has been stagnant for the past decade. Ironically, in the age of artificial intelligence, a recent report by Australia's Productivity Commission says that across the OECD, growth in GDP per hour worked was lower in the decade to 2016 than in any decade from 1950.[31] The report went on to suggest that healthcare could play a leading role in improving national performance and highlights a change in thinking about productivity.

It says the emphasis has shifted from the need to produce goods more cheaply to improving human capital—the knowledge, skills, and work practices of staff—and delivering more efficient and effective health, education, and related services. The report recognizes that Australia is now predominantly a service economy and that healthcare is a both a clinical service and a significant economic driver. Like other OECD countries, healthcare represents a growing share of the Australian workforce, growing from 1.1 million to 1.6 million—13.3% of the total—in the decade to 2017. Employment in retail, mining, and manufacturing has remained static. Significantly, the productivity report concludes that improving the effectiveness of the healthcare workforce 'would bring welfare gains for the individuals concerned, savings for the health system and gains for the economy more broadly'.

Change is a human contact sport

The increased motivation and improved performance management of the health workforce is one of the most neglected areas in health practice today. The trapped potential of millions of people across health systems is enormous. In nearly every conference I speak at, I ask the audience what percentage of their staff have meaningful objective-setting and appraisals which are aligned with their team's or organization's objectives. You may be shocked to learn that only one-fifth to one-third put their hands up. How can people deliver compassionate care if they are not cared for too?

As the Chartered Institute of Personnel and Development stresses, there is a consensus among academics and practitioners that performance appraisal can encourage a range of organizational outcomes including task performance, productivity, loyalty, satisfaction, and commitment. Yet, ironically, the special status of caregivers is often used as an excuse to ignore standard management techniques that work perfectly well elsewhere. Healthcare professionals should be given more responsibility and accept greater accountability for what they do.

If change is a human contact sport, then we had better contact human beings. Organizational charts often juxtapose organizational health (so-called softer measures such as culture, staff well-being, and organizational development) with organizational performance (the hard metrics of activity, margins, profit and loss, or shareholder return). While you can always perform better on one than the other for a limited time, in the long run the best organizations seek a balance. The same should run true for hospitals and health systems.

Health organizations can become substantially more efficient and effective just through smarter objectives and better appraisal, management, and staff development. As noted in Value Walks, the KPMG International report in 2016, there are five characteristics that separate great health employers from the good and the bad: a strategic focus on value for patients, empowered staff, process redesign, innovative use of technology, and the management of staff performance. Given the looming workforce shortage, we need to broaden the skill base for health and care staff, encourage their flexibility, and reduce costly demarcations that do not serve patients' interests. In other industries the war for talent is seen as mission critical; the same urgency needs to be applied on an industrial scale in healthcare.

Inverting and reimagining the pyramid of care

The clinical hierarchy of doctors, nurses, allied health professionals, and care assistants has remained largely unchanged for a century or more, and most spending on education, training, and development of healthcare workers is focused at the top of the skills pyramid. This fails to reflect the rapid rise of chronic conditions for which lower-skilled care workers, alongside devices, technology, and algorithms, can provide substantial levels of support as well as encourage a significant degree of self-management.

To be clear, I am certainly not arguing that clinical staff should get less attention, but given the impending workforce shortages there is a compelling opportunity for untapped labour sources to enter the healthcare workforce. We will talk later about patients and the part they can play in leveraging our productive capability, but we should also mobilize at scale people with basic secondary education qualifications, the underemployed, and the unemployed. These people tend to live and work in the communities that need their help.

My solution is to invert the traditional thinking about investment in skills and create a large cadre of care workers that today might be called care assistants. Instead of recruiting, training, developing, and paying at different rates and various ways, employers and educators should come together across health, social care, and human services. As I shall describe later, the most radical approach to changing the pyramid of care I have seen is Buurtzorg, the home care provider in the Netherlands, which supports tens of thousands of people through self-directing nurses, each providing a wide range of skills from basic to advanced, backed by a flat management structure.

Within our grasp

What could be more important to human beings and nations than the health of the world's citizens? Health, and how a country cares for its people, is a hallmark of a civilized society. I was a member of the NHS Management Board that published the first Constitution for the NHS back in 2008 (to celebrate its sixtieth birthday). It stated that 'the NHS belongs to the people and exists to improve our health and well-being, supporting us to keep mentally and physically well, to get better when we are ill and, when we cannot recover, to stay as well as we can to the end of our lives. It works at the limits of science—bringing the highest levels of human knowledge and skill to save lives and improve health. It touches our lives at times of basic human need, when care and compassion are what matters most'. These are noble goals for any country, and they are within our grasp.

All of this sounds fine on an objective, detached level but as we all know, health and healthcare matters most when it's personal. My world was shaken when I discovered, quite by chance, that I had prostate cancer at the age of 42. Ten years on, and thanks to a radical prostatectomy provided by the NHS, performed by a German surgeon and cared for by a charge nurse from the Philippines and a British general practitioner, I am fortunate to be able to enjoy my life, my children, my community, and a job that takes me to every corner of our amazing planet. Without the globalization of science, health workers, and their skills, where would I be? Where would we all be?

Chapter 2

Productivity—health and wealth

Nobel Laureate economist Paul Krugman said 'productivity isn't everything, but in the long run it is almost everything'.[1] Productivity is the ultimate engine of economic growth in the global economy, yet health leaders have been sheepish, even scornful, of debating it.

This has hampered investment and allowed national decision-makers to get away with tactical, short-term, feast-and-famine funding decisions which have hindered the ability of healthcare to make a substantial and sustainable contribution to national wealth creation through raised productivity. Healthcare, with its wonderful improvements in life expectancy, can present a powerful moral, ethical, and social argument for its contribution to human development and achievement, but some health professionals believe this argument is so axiomatic that debate should stop there. This is unwise.

Productivity is about working smarter, not harder. It reflects our ability to produce more outputs (goods and services) from defined inputs (labour and capital). Productivity is improved through better education and skills, innovation, technological advances, improved infrastructure, and enhanced or disruptive business models—and, of course, better leadership. It is cultivated through the global exchange of ideas, labour, and capital and was the main source of economic prosperity and well-being throughout the twentieth century.

Innovations from the wheel to the steam engine, from electrification to digitization, have led to outstanding improvements in the production of goods and services which have raised living standards and life satisfaction. The Organisation for Economic Co-operation and Development (OECD) notes that the large differences in income per capita between and across countries mostly reflect differences in labour productivity. While global productivity has slowed somewhat since the global financial crisis of 2008, it is still expected to be the main driver of economic growth this century. Health policies that ignore this do so at their peril.

We should not confuse productivity gains with efficiencies or cost reduction. Productivity deals with the time to produce a good or service, whereas efficiency looks at the cost. Put another way, productivity is all about the rate at which output is achieved and efficiency the cost of doing so. This chapter is certainly not arguing for major cost efficiencies. We have tried that in the English National Health Service (NHS) and saw a cherished national institution momentarily knocked to its knees during the winter of 2017–2018.

Global productivity trends

Productivity across all industries has risen by around 2% per year since the Second World War. Research into health productivity is patchy but the most optimistic estimate is an increase of around 0.9% per year. But against this global improvement, commentators such as Bob Kocher in the *Harvard Business Review* suggest American healthcare labour productivity has historically declined at a rate of 0.6% per year.

A recent European Policy Brief compared health productivity in Germany, Spain, Hungary, and the UK. As always, comparisons are difficult, but it appears that from 2003 to 2009 productivity declined by 1.5% per year in Hungary and 1% in Spain, while it improved by 0.7% in the UK and 2% in Germany.[2] In a separate report, the University of York suggested NHS productivity growth was higher, at around 1.4% per annum (2004/5–2013/14) but a more recent report from the ONS puts it lower at 1.25%. Over 20 years, that equates to 25% productivity growth with 3% reported for 2017.[3] On the other side of the world meanwhile, the New Zealand Productivity Commission says its health productivity grew by 0.9%.[4]

Generalizations in this under-researched area of healthcare are problematic but it is fairly safe to assume that, globally, healthcare productivity growth is about half that of other sectors in the economy. When this is combined with the fact that, over the past 60 years, health spending has risen in OECD countries by an average of 2% more than gross domestic product (GDP) growth, it is easy to see why some question the long-term sustainability of healthcare. This argument can and must be refuted but health leaders need to engage seriously with the productivity debate to protect existing gains and secure future progress. For health is wealth. Investments in health can dramatically improve productivity, living standards, wages, and national economic performance.

The United Kingdom has a chronic productivity problem, lagging towards the bottom of G7 countries. Indeed, in 2016 chancellor Philip Hammond proclaimed that 'the productivity gap is well-known but shocking nonetheless. It takes a German worker four days to produce what we make in five, which means, in turn, that too many British workers work longer hours for lower pay than their counterparts'. The government published a 15-point plan and announced a four-year, £31 billion commitment to a National Productivity Investment Fund.[5] The NHS did not bid for, or receive, a single penny.

Like America and other developed countries, United Kingdom average real-term wages will not be any higher in 2022 than a year before the global financial crisis. Wage stagnation for a decade and a half is unprecedented and, as I have seen across continents, has certainly been felt by health workers as their wages have been suppressed at or below economic growth and price inflation.

Many commentators say a low-wage, low-skills economy thwarts productivity improvements because employers rely on cheap labour rather than make long-term investments in technology and equipment which ultimately enhance profitability, productivity, and wages. Who can take pride in wanting to be 'the sweat shop of the world'? Further, investments in infrastructure such as roads, railways, airports, and broadband all improve productivity, as does funding for research, education, training, and more agile vocational skills.

Improved management and better employee engagement increase motivation and productivity, while disruptive and superior business models, facilitated through innovation, adoption, and adaption increase competitive capability. Encouraging or incentivizing customers or end users to take over part of the production process itself (think online banking or the Amazon cashless supermarket) can also improve productivity. No wonder the UK chancellor declared 'if we raised our productivity by just 1% every year, within a decade we would add £250 billion to the size of our economy; £9,000 for every household in Britain'. This would translate into a substantial prize for every country.

Healthcare's role in economic growth

Health can play a more prominent role in improving national productivity. The deal is strikingly simple: health funding and health salaries to be linked to productivity increases in return for serious long-term economic investment in the areas which help healthcare drive national growth.

It is worth noting the commendable work of *The Lancet* and others in demonstrating how the pursuit of universal healthcare can enhance countries' economic performance (Fig. 2.1). Extending productive life plays an important role in nation-building, social cohesion, social mobility, and reducing inequalities. All these benefits can generate significant economic gains.

There is now a substantial body of literature supporting the view that increased healthcare coverage fuels economic growth through improved productivity and employment, better educational attainment, and increased protection from healthcare bills that push tens of millions into poverty each year and inhibit spending in other parts of the economy.

In recent years compelling analysis has demonstrated the importance of access to healthcare in a thriving economy. In 2013 a seminal review by a *Lancet* commission of leading economists found that approximately 11% of economic growth in low- and middle-income countries between 2000 and 2011 resulted from reduced mortality.[6]

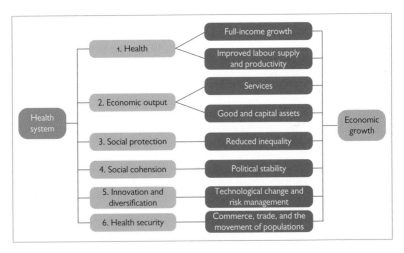

Fig. 2.1 Pathways to economic growth.
Reproduced with permission from Buchan, J. et al. (Eds). Health Employment and Economic Growth: An Evidence Base. Geneva, Switzerland: World Health Organization. Copyright © 2017 WHO.

But this number only captures the hard-edged economic impact. Taking into account the intrinsic benefits of better health, the overall gains are far greater. A more complete picture capturing the value of additional life years as well as the direct economic benefits is given in a country's 'full income'; the commission concluded that between 2000 and 2011, about 24% of the growth in full income in low-income and middle-income countries resulted from the value of additional life years gained. This relates to factors such as improved labour productivity (through longer and healthier lives and lower absenteeism), improved child health, and educational attainment, and the ratio of workers to dependents. They concluded that 'there is an enormous payoff from investing for health'. Over 20 years the return on health investment could be nine to one.

In my own team's work in the Bahamas, where KPMG helped develop the first phase of universal healthcare through the rollout of a primary care platform and a new National Health Insurance scheme, we calculated that economic growth would be 4.8% greater over 20 years through a reduction in catastrophic health costs and associated increases in discretionary spend in other parts of the economy, reduced absenteeism, and more working hours at higher productivity. The increase in economic performance over 20 years is expected to be seven times higher than the cost of the policy.

Similarly, a 2004 study found that a one-year improvement in a population's life expectancy increases output by 4%.[7] In the Australian context, a recent study found that a 1% decrease in cancer mortality rates would result in a 1.6% increase in GDP per capita.[8] Put simply, an increase in health status raises investment in human capital and spurs economic growth.

The fallacy of poor healthcare productivity

Before we turn to ways in which healthcare productivity can be boosted, it is worth acknowledging why healthcare is unlikely to match the productivity gains of other sectors. Traditional economic analysis of productivity has clear data on inputs, outputs, and outcomes. But healthcare is different. Hospitals are not factories. There are tomes of dense, dry papers which explain why, but the arguments are essentially twofold.

First, healthcare is a human contact service industry which relies on human beings caring for other human beings. Second, because of the highly personal nature of care and the multiplicity of causes, treatments, and outcomes, measuring quantitative outputs (consultations, ambulatory procedures, operations, and so on) and qualitative outcomes in a meaningful way is problematic. This difficulty is exacerbated by the paucity and unreliability of long-term clinical outcome data. For example, a new procedure or medical device may improve quality of life and reduce readmissions many years later, but it is all but impossible to account for this in the numbers.

Across most developed health economies, care is labour intensive. The King's Fund in London estimates that staff account for around 70% of a typical hospital's costs[9] and this proportion has grown over time—even as other industries' labour costs have fallen dramatically. We have already noted that cost and price pressures have been stronger in the health sector than the rest of the economy while productivity is lower. In 2016, the UK Office for Budget Responsibility's report on the fiscal sustain-ability of health said the reason for this was the 'Baumol cost disease' (not a flattering name in any situation) where 'real wages in the healthcare sector have to keep pace with the rest of the economy in order to attract and retain staff but slower product-ivity growth means that additional input would be needed to achieve the required improvement in care per person. As a result, the cost of health services will rise relative to other sectors of the economy'.[10] So, there we have it.

Except that this theory does not explain productivity variations between hos-pitals in the same area, region, or country or across health systems on the same continent. For example, an excellent report produced in the United Kingdom by the Royal College of Ophthalmologists and British Orthopaedic Association concluded that 'if every NHS provider followed the good operational practices adopted by the highest performers at each stage of their elective ophthalmology and ortho-paedic care pathways, they could save 13–20% of today's spending on planned care in these two specialities'.[11] These two account for around one-third of NHS elective care spend.

Other industrial and service sectors suffer the same malaise. An OECD report on the future of productivity says labour productivity at the global frontier (the best performing manufacturing companies across the world) increased at an average an-nual rate of 3.5% compared with average labour productivity growth of just 0.5% for non-frontier firms.[12] This gap is even more pronounced in the services sector. The central cause of variation across and within sectors is the ability to innovate, adapt, and adopt. The crucial issue therefore, is one of diffusion.

World-class innovation

This point is beautifully illustrated in a recent King's Fund report on the adoption and spread of innovation in the NHS.[13] They rightly state that entrepreneurship is alive and well in the NHS but point to a chronic problem in wider adoption of innovative ideas and practices. Investment in research and development stood at £1.2 billion in 2017 but only £50 million was dedicated to spreading good practice. This represents less than 0.1% of total NHS spending. The report says this small fraction means 'the NHS's operating units will struggle to adopt large numbers of innovations and rapidly improve productivity'.

The report claims some private sector multinationals set aside up to 25% of turn-over to promote innovations. While I think this sounds too high, I can certainly con-firm that KPMG spends proportionately more time and money than most health systems making sure best practice and knowledge is diffused quickly and evenly to maintain competitive edge.

I have seen outstanding examples of innovative, highly productive, patient-centred clinical service models all over the world. I will outline just a few to highlight what could be achieved if the rest engaged with the best.

In Bangladesh, Norwegian telecoms company Telenor has developed a phone-based care service which has attracted millions of users because of its low costs, high quality, and great access. They researched the most common unmet needs and dis-covered that consumers wanted to speak to health professionals they could trust at a time which suited them and without the financial burden typically associated with quality healthcare in this low-income country.

Working through Grameen Phone as distributor they developed Tonic, a digital healthcare service providing affordable, comprehensive healthcare to its subscribers. Paying a monthly, tiered subscription to meet different needs, patients speak directly to doctors and other clinicians to get advice, prescriptions, and medication. Over four million people joined in the first nine months. Over 70% of all calls and enquiries are dealt with on the phone or internet, with artificial intelligence algorithms guiding consultations. Think of the global productivity gains if 70% of primary care appointments could take place on the phone or internet. The phone company has also developed Bangladesh's first portable health record.

Critics may claim that Bangladesh is atypical, but this would be wrong. In Mexico, MedicalHome provides telephone-based advice and care to over five million people. For a monthly enrolment fee of $5 charged to the phone bill, members can access doctors 24/7. Diagnosis is based on standardized clinical protocols developed by the Cleveland Clinic. Members have access to a network of 6,000 physicians and approximately two-thirds of all cases are dealt with on the phone.

Similarly, the Californian not-for-profit healthcare organization Kaiser Permanente has developed an online communication and consultation service between patients and their clinicians. Over 65% of consultations and enquiries take place this way, dramatically improving access, satisfaction, and quality. I was recently in Oakland, California, and asked Kaiser doctors whether they would ever like to go back to solely traditional face-to-face consultations. They said that neither patients nor professionals would want it that way.

In the Bronx, New York, the Montefiore Medical Center has used remote patient monitoring to reduce hospital admissions for elderly patients by over 30%. I saw how decent information technology helped dedicated clinical teams provide responsive, sensitive care to patients living in hard-pressed communities, and thought that if they can do it there, we can do it anywhere.

In Israel Clalit, the leading health maintenance organization (HMO) uses artificial intelligence algorithms to manage population health by uploading individual clinical risk indicators every day and deploying clinical teams to patients deemed at risk before illness flares up. Having seen it first hand, I believe this anticipatory healthcare is the new gold standard in population health management and primary care. It reduces costs significantly and is dramatically more productive and efficient.

Information technology is essential to integrated care. In Valencia, Spain, the integrated care system uses clinical protocols between primary and secondary care to manage both flow and demand in a single health system. Independent analysis suggests it is over 20% more efficient and productive than other, uncoordinated Spanish health systems.

In India, a combination of clinical process redesign, standardization, role flexibility, and low-cost technology has allowed hospital operators to deliver care at one-fifth the cost in the West. The Aravind Eye Hospital, founded by Dr Govindappa Venkataswamy in 1976 with the mission to eradicate blindness in India, was inspired by the McDonalds business model to deliver consistently high-quality, low-cost ophthalmic services in the most productive way. The hospitals have a wonderful and curious culture which combines six sigma process improvement and spirituality with a start-up mentality and an unswerving service focus supported by outstanding teamwork and clinician communication.

I have seen how the Narayana Health hospital group in India has taken cardiac care clinical standardization to new levels, producing outcomes comparable with the Cleveland Clinic, while my good friend Dr Prathap Reddy, Chairman of the Apollo Hospital Group, has taken telemedicine to impressive heights. Around 80% of the Indian population lives in rural areas but over 80% of doctors practise in cities. Apollo has developed a state-of-the-art telehealth service which provides for all parts of India (and now other parts of the world) at a fraction of the cost of traditional bricks and mortar. Quality, access, efficiency, and productivity have all improved.

On seeing this system in action former US President Bill Clinton said: 'This is a very wonderful contribution to the healthcare of the people who live in rural villages and I hope that people all over the world will follow your lead.' We are still waiting.

Across the world there are thousands more examples of isolated excellence. The cyberpunk novelist William Gibson once said that 'the future is already here, it's just not evenly distributed'. This certainly applies to healthcare. In later chapters we will explore the huge potential of the workforce, technology, artificial intelligence, government legislation and action, public–private partnerships, consumer co-production, and more to drive massive improvements in productivity. It is abundantly clear that gains between 10% and 30% are achievable just through scalable care model innovation and business model disruption.

Throughout my travels I have had the opportunity to engage with some of the world's outstanding healthcare leaders and teams, and several themes consistently emerge. High-productivity health systems reimagine care delivery through the creative application of technology and artificial intelligence. The application of technology is successful because they take time and effort to understand user or consumer behaviour and encourage greater co-production with staff.

Lean organizations standardize wherever possible and give clinicians the freedom to act, but have loose/tight mechanisms for responsibility and accountability fostered through a collaborative, restless, and enquiring culture. This enables them to challenge traditional professional assumptions and skill the workforce appropriately, allowing a more permissive and inclusive appreciation of the role patients and carers can play in co-producing healthcare.

Successful organizations often have an open approach to alliances and partnerships which can include the use of non-health assets such as telecommunications, retailers, and technology companies. They are not afraid to fail fast and learn quickly and have a transparently fair way of dealing with mishaps and setbacks.

The size of the productivity prize

I was a member of the World Economic Forum Health Council from 2014 to 2018. Recent McKinsey research for it concluded that scaling up improvements to primary care systems (like MedicalHome in Mexico) could reduce visits by 30%, while standardizing care pathways for planned and elective admissions (like the NHS in England or private hospital operators in India) could yield productivity gains of 20%. Adopting and adapting integrated care models found in Spain or Israel could produce efficiencies of at least 10% and the subsequent management of long-term, chronic diseases could conservatively improve cost management by 15%.[14]

The authors concluded that 'taking these four aspects together, we calculate that successful implementation could lead to a 16% reduction in healthcare spending'.

This is even before we look at opportunities for reengineering productivity gains in administrative and business systems. The blockchain revolution, robotics, and artificial intelligence are already automating routine functions. In this light, I believe the productivity prize is closer to 20% if sensible long-term investments are made and implementation is planned, phased, and resourced well.

If you are not convinced by the arguments I have rehearsed, consider this quote from the New Zealand Productivity Commission: 'Not only will the demand for key public services increase but we can also expect growth in the aggregate labour force to slow. The implication is that public sector managers can expect their services to face greater demand as input growth becomes more constrained, and so they are going to need to increasingly focus on lifting productivity.'

Does anyone have a better Plan B? The following chapters outline numerous ways in which our workforce can be more productive, allowing our health systems to contribute to national and global wealth creation and, by doing so, enjoy the rewards they richly deserve.

Chapter 3

India—the march of Modicare

I arrived in Delhi the week after Prime Minister Narendra Modi announced plans to extend universal healthcare to half a billion people from the poorest 100 million families in India. Claiming it to be the largest single move to universal care in history, the plans are breathtaking in scale, especially given the poor starting base. Apocryphally, it has been claimed it would take India nearly a century to train all the health workers it needs, so necessity will need be the mother of innovation. But India does have some success to build on. 'Jugaad' is a Hindi word which means solving complex problems with ingeniously simple solutions, and it has certainly been applied to standardization and skills shifting in health which have enabled millions of patients to receive good-quality care at a fraction of the cost in the West.

The enormity of 'Modicare' represents a proud moment in Indian history and a firm statement of ambition. As finance minister Arun Jaitley said in his Budget speech, 'India cannot realize its demographic dividend without its citizens being healthy'. But the government is belatedly realizing that one of the biggest challenges among many in delivering Modicare will be securing a workforce of sufficient scale and quality, which meets the needs of rural as well as urban areas.

Modern doctors, traditional healers

Developing a workforce strategy is not helped by poor data about its current resources. With a population of 1.3 billion, estimates suggest a target of 4.6 million skilled healthcare workers. The World Health Organization (WHO) believes there are currently fewer than 2.1 million—less than half what is needed. To complicate estimates, this includes 'AYUSH' practitioners—Ayurveda, Yoga, Unani, Siddha, and Homeopathy—traditional Indian treatments still practised and respected alongside qualified, allopathic doctors, nurses, midwives, and paramedics.

The many informal health workers confuse these figures further, as up to half of those working as allopathic doctors in rural areas are in truth 'registered medical practitioners' with no formal medical qualifications and high numbers of 'quacks'. Figure 3.1 illustrates the wide disparities in education among health workers.

The need to accommodate the traditional AYUSH approach is underlined by the profound imbalance in access across this vast country. The healthcare workforce simply is not where it is needed. Nearly 60% of health workers live in urban areas, which account for only 28% of the population. About 59% of urban allopathic doctors are medically qualified, compared with 19% in rural areas.[1]

This leaves swathes of the population—particularly in rural areas—dependent on traditional treatments and unqualified staff. Overall you have a 1 in 10 chance of walking into a primary health centre and finding a medically qualified doctor, with

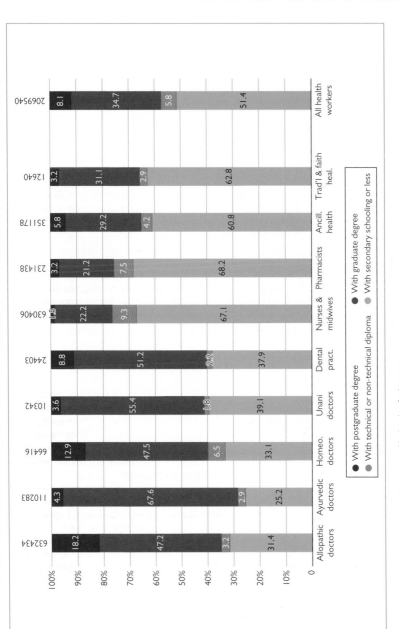

Fig. 3.1 Health workers by category: disaggregated by levels of education.

just with just 0.8 physicians per 1,000 inhabitants in 2016 compared with 2.5 in the United States and 3.2 in Europe, placing it among the lowest ratios globally.[2]

Against this profoundly challenging backdrop it is not surprising that many medically qualified doctors take the opportunity to emigrate, with nearly half of medical college graduates going to work overseas, mostly in the United States. It is difficult to establish how many eventually come back, returning as 'superstar doctors' with respected foreign medical credentials and commanding considerably higher private incomes. Nonetheless, shortages of doctors in developed countries coupled with better postgraduate training and career opportunities create a substantial drain on the number of practitioners.

Yet the population has adjusted to this reality, with patients reporting similar degrees of trust in AYUSH practitioners as qualified doctors. The challenge is therefore striking a balance between moving away from AYUSH practitioners and informal health workers providing nearly all care in more rural settings, while recognizing that without engaging them in some way there will not be anything like enough staff. Recognizing this, the government is planning an Allied and Healthcare Professional Council Bill, which will lead to more than 55 types of allied and other health workers receiving professional recognition, career pathways, and meaningful employment.

Tamil Nadu is one state that has made a provision for education of physicians and nurses in the private sector and worked to put incentives and policies in place to attract and retain staff. In return for this education, professionals have three years of mandatory rural service to help balance the urban and rural divide. Unlike Tamil Nadu, most states in India do not have a workforce policy to ensure that doctors are being rotated between rural and urban positions. This has created a perception for Indian doctors that while rural service is a much-needed service to their people and their country, they have no hope of leaving that post with credentials and documented work experience that could allow them to work in an urban setting again—a huge disincentive to taking up these posts.

Reaching the villages

In such a large country, reorganizing care to put the right people in the right place will clearly be an important part of future healthcare worker management in implementing Modicare, but this alone will be insufficient, not to say unrealistic. While most states offer higher salaries for public sector doctors working in rural areas, this has done little to address the problem at the scale required. Whole new ways of working will be needed, from reshaping the workforce through to public–private partnerships.

A recent focus on human resources by the Ministry of Health has sought to set out what new ways of working might look like. Acknowledging the shortages of trained doctors, the logistics of serving 600,000 villages, and the existing AYUSH and non-trained medical workers already serving these has provided a starting point for thinking about new models of healthcare delivery. In these settings not only would it be difficult to find a doctor to serve the community, but that doctor would not necessarily have the trust of the local community compared with a long-standing AYUSH practitioner. Instead, basic trainees—potentially drawn from AYUSH practitioners—are estimated to be able to care for 70% of primary care problems in these settings, allowing for greater emphasis on strengthening appropriate referral pathways onwards from rural care.

This rural care is divided into three tiers. The first tier are subcentres, operated by trained health workers and auxiliary nurse midwives. The second are primary health centres, supported by an allopathic doctor, paramedics, and other staff. The third tier is the community health centre, where the required staff include a surgeon, a physician, a gynaecologist, a paediatrician, paramedics, and other staff. While the classification and expected staffing provides a useful start, understaffing in these centres remains hugely problematic.

Central to much of this work around new workforce models has been a mapping exercise to classify the many different healthcare work roles in India into 'skilled', 'allied', and 'healthcare'. A lack of transparency about what these different groups do has previously hindered planning. Understanding this better has led to opportunities to deliver task-based training. This is particularly relevant to the 'skilled' and 'allied' levels, where providing an aspirational in-job training route for career progression is an important step in aiding recruitment and retention.

This innovative work has not been without controversy, and dominant professional groups have been reluctant to give up any powers. In 2018, a government bill to address the severe workforce shortages by allowing traditional AYUSH practitioners and informal health workers to practice 'Western' medicine after completing a bridging course was branded as 'disastrous . . . anti-patient and anti-doctor' by the Indian Medical Association, culminating in over 300,000 doctors striking. Although many see this task-shifting as an essential short-term remedy to deal with workforce shortages, it seems that a strong medical profession will continue to obstruct it.

Unfortunately reports of widespread corruption continue to undermine this position; from selling seats for postgraduate medical training to the ease with which basic healthcare worker qualifications and even fake medical degrees can be bought by 'quacks', corruption is a reality across the healthcare workforce in India.

The need for higher quality

But India's healthcare workforce problems are not only a matter of numbers and distributional imbalance. Long-standing problems of poor career structures, weak management and supervision, an inefficient mix of skills and inadequate training are all signs of neglect around workforce policy and practice. With over 70 types of healthcare worker and little regulation, there are significant opportunities for improving oversight and care quality. What regulation does exist lacks teeth, with little focus on quality and standards. While addressing these issues might seem an obvious course, considerable resistance has stalled progress to date. Initiatives in this area lack private sector support, because they are concerned that standard-setting through accreditation, certification, and assessment would result in having to pay staff more.

With an under-resourced public health system, the private sector has grown to become the dominant employer with 70% of all health workers (although the distinction between public and private sectors is often blurred, particularly in states that allow public doctors to run private clinics). Despite this dominance, nurses and midwives often prefer public sector employment to private because of better job security and pay and fixed working hours.

Recruitment rules and standards for healthcare workers also vary dramatically between the private and public, as do rules around continuous in-service training. Given the much larger patient load in the public facilities, the average medical, allied, or nursing caregiver there tends to develop greater expertise than their private sector counterpart. Yet patient costs are higher in the private sector, with no guarantee of clinical quality. Instead, the service quality—which tends to be much higher in the private sector—becomes the factor on which the average consumer decides whether the healthcare they are getting is 'good' or 'bad'. If universal healthcare is to become a reality, the chasm between the private and public sectors in quality, costs, and access will need to be addressed though robust regulation.

Standardized excellence

A small number of private healthcare providers in India are combining American assembly-line methods with Japanese lean management techniques and the 'jugaad' approach of finding simple solutions to complex problems to deliver high-quality treatment at a fraction of Western costs.

Narayana Health runs multispecialty hospitals that exploit economies of scale at every opportunity to improve quality and reduce cost. Their largest facility is a 5,000 bed 'health city': a factory for cardiac surgery and cancer care with the fixed costs spread over as many patients as possible. They further leverage scale by centralizing support services across the network—teleradiology is done in a single hub in Bangalore, and purchasing is unified across the chain. Narayana's goal is to perform heart operations at a cost of $800 per patient. With what they have done so far, they may well achieve it.

Two other world-leading private providers—Apollo Hospital and Aravind Eye Care—follow a similar model of using volume to increase quality while decreasing cost. A major part of the formula is leveraging the scarce professional skills of doctors to the maximum degree possible; they only work on tasks that require a doctor, with other activities like pre and postoperative care delegated to task-specialist support workers. Aravind doctors perform 1,000 to 1,400 eye surgeries a year compared with an average of 400 among US doctors.[3] This is achieved by making sure doctors only do what only doctors can do.

Many expected this production line method to result in worse outcomes, but both Aravind and Apollo demonstrate equivalent (and in some cases better) outcomes than is typical in the West because of the close relationship between volume and quality in surgery—the more someone does a procedure, the better they are at it.[4]

Conclusion

There is a pride in 'Made in India', but there have been many false dawns for universal healthcare before. This time I am more hopeful this 'kaleidoscope' country will arrive at a unique solution for its complex healthcare workforce problems. Nonetheless, better geographic redistribution and strategic planning of the healthcare workforce is going to be key. It is important that the government urgently gets to grips with developing a national healthcare workforce plan, with a place for all care practitioners with the right supervision and guidance. If Indian people trust these traditional providers already, then working with them in new ways, within a better regulated system, to help them work to their fullest potential is surely the right step to take if the promise of Modicare is to be delivered to India's people. With the scale and geographical spread of workforce needed, this is the only practical solution to the colossal workforce challenge of Modicare.

But the most impressive innovators in India are showing the world just how far standardization and skill shifting in pursuit of low-cost, high-quality care can be taken. Developing technicians with huge expertise and experience in a narrowly defined task—while liberating doctors to do what only they can do—could be the beginning of a revolution in the delivery of complex care. The performance management which accompanies this approach enforces high standards of delivery and accountability, while the astonishing levels of productivity and the quality of the outcomes provide a motivating environment in which to work. We should be intrigued by the possibilities of harnessing non-traditional healthcare worker roles to deliver better care at low cost while admiring what can be achieved through excellent care process redesign.

Chapter 4

Israel—start-up nation

The Israeli health system has always fascinated me as one of the best-kept secrets in healthcare. While many people talk about a primary care-led health system, they seldom achieve it. Israel seems to be almost unique in this respect, making it happen with four health maintenance organizations (HMOs) providing citizens with both choice and comprehensive cover.

Primary and community care spend first exceeded that of secondary and acute care 20 years ago, but it has taken time. Its origins can be traced back to 1911 when an orchard worker had his arm severed and 150 immigrant workers joined together to form a mutual aid healthcare organization called Clalit, a non-governmental, non-profit entity. They knew that to help themselves they had to help each other, and Clalit is now the largest HMO in Israel with 14 hospitals and more than 1,200 primary and specialized clinics. The health system of Israel is not perfect but is highly innovative—not least in its use of patient information—and deserves attention.

Low cost, long life

For a modest 7.8% of GDP spent on healthcare the country delivers one of the highest life expectancies in the OECD.[1] Although Israelis themselves sometimes perceive a health system in difficulty, the population enjoys comparatively good health built on foundations of strong efforts in public health and progressive primary care services. The sophisticated system is state run, with mandatory health insurance provided by one of four HMOs: Clalit and Maccabi, the two largest which serve most of the population, and the smaller Leumit and Meuhedet.

Severe shortages

On the surface current medical staffing levels compare reasonably well with other developed countries, with 3.4 physicians per 1,000 in 2016, giving 35,000 physicians serving a population of 8.7 million. But looking behind these numbers it is clear that trouble is looming. They are potentially flattered by both poor data and the historical immigration of large numbers of doctors from the Soviet Union in the 1990s. As Figure 4.1 illustrates, overseas trained doctors make up the majority now practising in Israel, but many are nearing retirement, with some 70% of licensed doctors aged 45 or over, and it is increasingly common for retirement age physicians to be asked to carry on working. Given Israel's dependence on a strong primary care system, there is concern that shortages are particularly effecting family physicians. Here, more than 40% are over 60 years old.[2]

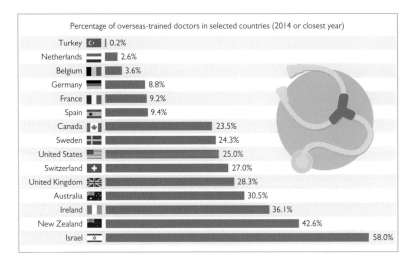

Percentage of overseas-trained doctors in selected countries (2014 or closest year)

Country	Percentage
Turkey	0.2%
Netherlands	2.6%
Belgium	3.6%
Germany	8.8%
France	9.2%
Spain	9.4%
Canada	23.5%
Sweden	24.3%
United States	25.0%
Switzerland	27.0%
United Kingdom	28.3%
Australia	30.5%
Ireland	36.1%
New Zealand	42.6%
Israel	58.0%

Fig. 4.1 The countries with the most foreign-trained doctors.

Reproduced from McCarthy, N. The Countries With The Most Foreign-Trained Doctors. Statista. Oct 5, 2015. Copyright © 2015 Statista. Available at https://www.statista.com/chart/3849/the-countries-with-the-most-foreign-trained-doctors/

The number of Israeli physicians emigrating has also increased, many citing burnout and poor pay. There is a particular shortage of anaesthesiologists—over the past decade around a fifth have emigrated.

Even with a new fifth medical school recently opening, and continued immigration (Aliyah) of doctors—895 in 2017[3]—the estimated future physician demand seems unlikely to be met without changes. This is exacerbated by what some have called a crisis in medical education, with historically low numbers of home-grown medical graduates compared with future needs, and the lowest among OECD countries as recently as 2013. The government is narrowing this gap, sharply increasing the number of graduate training places; in 2015, 1,280 graduates started, compared with 912 in 2010.

These shortages are compounded by issues with local Israeli students being rejected from medical school in place of foreign overseas graduates (primarily from the United States). These make up nearly 15% of medical school intakes, but may never ultimately practise in Israel.[4] The high fees charged to them may offer a perverse incentive for their enrolment, which are up to 14 times higher than an Israeli student's fees. A recent analysis suggested that the multiple players in the medical education sector—universities, the Council for Higher Education, the Health Ministry, and hospitals—hinder progress in addressing these issues, with none having overall responsibility.[5]

Estimates of physician shortages are hard to come by, because the Ministry of Health does not produce any, but reports of waiting times for some specialties reaching as high as two years provide evidence of a serious and growing problem. The lack of data has fed the debate about the severity of shortages, with the Israeli Medical Association talking about a crisis.[6]

Unlike most Western countries, physicians in Israel are not required to take a regular licensing examination to remain in practice. The number of registered doctors is therefore a poor indicator of the true workforce numbers, and recent research has suggested a significant shortfall compared with official figures, with only 74% of those registered actually working and only 80% of those under 70 even living in Israel. This work also made clear that new trainees are insufficient to replace retirees.[7]

The picture is even less flattering for nursing, with long-standing severe shortages; Israel falls well behind the OECD average of 9.0 nurses per 1,000 people, with just 4.9 nurses per 1,000 in 2015.[8] Shortages are particularly severe in some specialties, with child deaths in neonatal intensive care units being directly attributed to shortages.[9] Similar to physicians, the age of the nursing workforce is also a looming issue, with 60% of nurses aged over 45. Whereas immigrant doctors have traditionally supported the low physician numbers, this has not been the case for nursing staff, with high barriers and bureaucratic restrictions to registration being reported.[10]

Staffing concerns are not restricted to doctors and nurses. They are now spreading to allied healthcare workers, and in 2018 some 5,000 physiotherapists, dietitians, speech therapists, occupational therapists, and others began protesting at overwork and staff shortages.[11]

Policy and protest

The Israeli government is responding to these issues. While the majority of Israeli physicians historically trained abroad (coming either as immigrants, or returners who studied overseas),[12] the government has recognized the increasing need to secure the supply of locally trained doctors. Expansion of training places is ongoing, with plans for a further medical school still being debated, but doubtless more needs to be done. Following adverse press coverage around neonatal deaths a further 400 nursing school places were announced in 2017, through new training programmes and expansion of existing courses. Both the University of Haifa and Tel Aviv University now run a programme that allows those already possessing a bachelor's degree to receive a Bachelor of Arts degree in nursing in two-and-a-half years instead of four.[13]

Unfortunately, some of these workforce reforms are being met with resistance. After years of discussion, physician assistant roles have recently been created, with the first graduates starting work in 2017.[14] Initially limited to Israeli-trained paramedics and physician assistants already qualified overseas, the need for these has arisen primarily in emergency medicine as a result of staff shortages, but there are also roles in anaesthesiology and pathology.[15] The Israeli Medical Association opposed establishing a physician assistant profession, suggesting that the country 're-examine its investments into the existing physician professions'. Despite this, legislation was passed, although it will take time for the impact of this new cadre of health workers to be felt.

Similar efforts by the Health Ministry to integrate highly trained nurse practitioners into community clinics with expanded authority at Maccabi HMO led to over 400 doctors writing in protest. Their petition complained that nurse practitioners 'who, after very brief training, will be able to diagnose in an amateurish manner acute and chronic illness, to write prescriptions for a range of conditions, to refer patients for tests and specialists, to draw up treatment plans, to write medical directives and more' was a 'great danger' causing widespread chaos.

While careful integration with adequate training is prerequisite for both physician assistants and nurse practitioners, the use of both in other health systems under physician supervision has been hailed as a success, and Israel would benefit from studying how this has been achieved. As per elsewhere in the world, fear of change and protectionism has been faced down by sheer practical need.

Digital health nation

Israel, the original 'start-up nation', is famously described in Dan Senor and Saul Singer's book on Israel's economic success as having produced more start-up companies than many larger and more stable nations. Healthcare has benefited from this phenomenon, with over 400 companies working in it.

From telemedicine through to point-of-care advanced diagnostics and artificial intelligence, Israeli healthcare start-ups are having an impact well beyond the borders of Israel, with great potential for reducing inefficiencies and increasing workforce productivity at home and abroad. The scale and pace of work in this area is among some of the brightest examples I have seen across the world. This is helped by support from the Israeli Ministry of Health, who promote technological innovation and foster entrepreneurship through pilot programmes worth around US$29 million a year over five years.[16]

The largest sector focusses on developing personal health tools that can track conditions and assist in their management and support. Through patient activation and empowerment, it is hoped demand on the health system can be reduced, freeing up clinician time and resources and helping patients stay in the community. The second largest subsector is data and analytics, with companies working to develop tools to predict, prevent, and diagnose medical conditions.

All of the HMOs, especially Clalit and Maccabi, have research and innovation centres that examine new technologies to improve the efficiency and effectiveness. A recent example is Maccabi's development and validation of a predictive model for detection of colorectal cancer in primary care by analysis of blood counts.

The increasing interest in predictive healthcare is one of the reasons for Maccabitech establishing a biobank to store samples from Maccabi members. They will be used in medical research into advanced precision medicine.

Through a dedicated e-health division, Clalit provides m-health and e-health services to over 1.25 million unique patients monthly. Pioneering innovations include online personal health records allowing patients to book clinic visits, renew prescriptions, set text messaging medication reminders, and hold telehealth consultations—notably providing paediatric medical consultations via video conferencing for out-of-hours emergencies.[17] A study at Clalit evaluating the first seven years of this service including 595,000 consultation calls showed that the average time from referral to obtaining medical advice was 6.6 minutes.[18] Imagine how many unnecessary emergency department attendances by worried patients were avoided, not to mention the benefit of quick reassurance and advice where appropriate. The service is now being expanded to patients with congestive heart failure,[19] and could transform care of long-term conditions in the community.

Already many years ahead of other health systems internationally, Clalit recently announced another big step forward in remote consultations through a partnership with Israeli start-up TytoCare.[20] The company is pioneering technology to conduct medical examinations and telehealth services remotely through a compact handheld device, which will allow patients to perform their own basic examinations under remote guidance such as checking temperature, ears, throat, lungs, and heart. While still at the pilot stage, it offers huge potential for freeing up clinic space and time.

Meanwhile, Maccabi, the second largest health fund, recently launched an innovative free smartphone application in collaboration with K Health. Using algorithms to draw on anonymous information from tens of millions of visits to Maccabi family physicians since 1992, when their health records were first computerized, the application is designed to replace unreliable internet searches for medical information. Using deep machine learning to gather information from consultations in similar situations, the application acts as a personal medical assistant. While not intending to replace a medical consultation, it is hoped that improved information will enable patients to make more informed and timely decisions about accessing healthcare.

The cleverest part of the Israeli health system brings together all the patient data collected, and with all four HMOs storing digital records, Israel is a world leader at harnessing the value of data to drive health innovation. This is supported by the government, who recently announced $287 million (1 billion shekels) to launch a new national 'big data' health project which will allow companies to access it. This publicly funded resource is intended as an economic growth engine. From a workforce perspective it offers the opportunity to make a giant leap in developing and testing digital innovations on real clinical data to increase productivity. From augmented clinical decision-making to safe and reliable process automation, Israel is likely to grow its start-up nation reputation.

Conclusion

An integrated, primary care-led, low-cost health system supporting a high life expectancy is a major achievement. Its innovative and comprehensive approach to patient data, coupled with a culture of technological innovation, is an example from which to learn.

The challenge for Israel will be ensuring that the pace of their technological innovation is reflected in new models of care. To do this they need to increase staff numbers and break out of their highly traditional approach to clinical roles. It is ironic that this 'start-up' nation can lead the world in technological and digital innovation but could leave many traditional clinical demarcations untouched. While I have seen many digital incubator sites, especially around Tel Aviv, I have seen less multidisciplinary collaboration between the tech industry and healthcare, but this is developing.

On a more positive note, patients and the general public seem more accepting of digital solutions than many countries, and the sociology and psychology of this success merits further global attention.

Chapter 5

Entrepreneurial government— from under to oversupply

The paradox of the global healthcare workforce is that while it has never been more abundant, it has never been scarcer relative to future patient needs. As Figure 5.1 shows, this workforce has largely been resistant to economic cycles of boom and bust, and has even flourished, relatively speaking, during recessions. But demand for health workers has surpassed our capacity to supply them and it has never been more important for governments to be progressive, agile, and courageous in tackling the looming crisis.

I have always believed that a thriving healthcare industry can improve national wealth and health. Not enough people appreciate the benefits of a well-resourced, trained, and motivated health workforce to society and the economy. Staff have been seen as a cost rather than an investment, resulting in poor workforce planning locally, nationally, and internationally. Traditional 'pool and flow' models, with images of a plentiful lake of workforce supply spontaneously finding its way down the natural tributaries of healthcare provision, are detached from wider societal, technological, and demographic changes. Unless governments reimagine their role in ensuring a healthy demand and supply of health workers, they risk undermining the contribution healthcare makes to the economy and individual well-being.

Supply, demand, and planning

Across the Organisation for Economic Co-operation and Development (OECD), the functioning of the labour market for health workers—for good or ill—is characterized by strong government interventions affecting both supply and demand.

On the demand side, we know that most health spending in nearly all OECD countries is publicly funded. Even in the United States, public spending on healthcare stands at $4,197 per head (the third highest) against an OECD average of $3,677.[1] Allocation of that public spending through reimbursement mechanisms affects demand for different types of health professionals. Governments operating any form of national health insurance scheme also determine demand by translating what might otherwise have been unmet need into a funded service. A range of other government policies affect demand for healthcare workers, including care quality standards, system efficiency, and the focus on prevention.

Governments have traditionally concentrated on supply side initiatives. Supply side forces include education and training, regulation, pay and pensions, as well as labour emigration and immigration policies. Most workforce plans concentrate on the

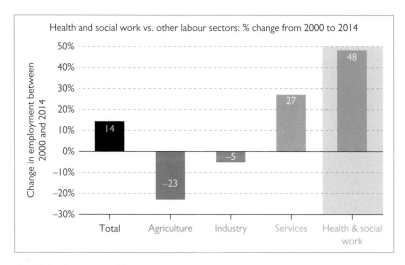

Fig. 5.1 Employment in health sector is growing.
Reproduced with permission from Campbell, J. Stress-testing our health systems – how prepared are we for the health workforce challenge? Salzburg, Austria: World Health Organization. Copyright 2018 © WHO.

minutiae of professional demarcations and numbers, reinforced through education, training, and regulation.

However, governments vary widely in the extent to which they accurately, actively, and iteratively plan their workforces. Countries such as the Netherlands have structured, sophisticated workforce modelling programmes. Others, such as the United Kingdom, are more fragmented. The Heath Foundation estimates that UK workforce planning involves 40 national statutory bodies, 15 royal colleges, 18 trade unions, and over 100 professional bodies—and that is before you add in hundreds of employers across health and social care. If you wanted to make sure nothing changed, this would be the way to do it.

National norms

Healthcare systems and governments seem to take for granted a rather random set of national norms for working hours, retirement age, rates of female participation in the workforce, and the proportion of health staff as a share of total employment. These norms place an artificial constraint on the capacity of the health workforce to meet demand. Looking at Figure 5.2 next, which highlights the wide variations between OECD countries, several conclusions can be drawn.

Until recently OECD retirement ages, which vary greatly, remained stubbornly fixed despite substantial improvements in lifespan. But since the 2008 financial crash most OECD countries have implemented or planned retirement age increases. Some self-employed doctors have chosen to delay their retirement plans because

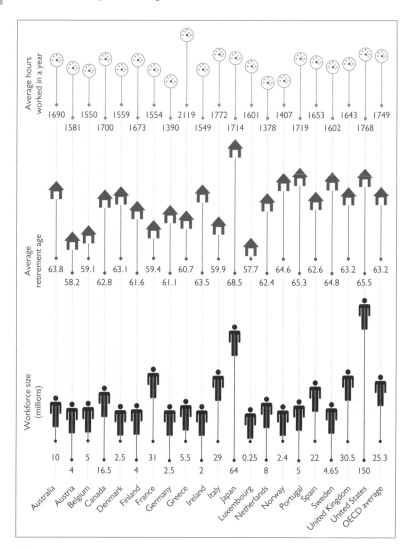

Fig. 5.2 The average number of hours worked per year and the average effective retirement age of countries compared by workforce.

of a fall in the value of pensions, investments, and property. Ironically, in the United Kingdom, where self-employed general practitioners enjoy the benefits of a state-funded pension, the reverse is true; doctors have been retiring earlier, as soon as their taxable pension pots have hit the maximum—a clear case of the left hand not knowing what the right hand is doing when it comes to workforce policy.

The impact of extending retirement ages is significant. The Netherlands' Advisory Committee on Medical Manpower Planning worked out that if the doctors who wanted to postpone retirement and work two years longer were able to do so, the total supply of doctors would grow by 4% between 2006 and 2030 instead of falling 1%. Similarly, the OECD estimates that the 2010 reforms to French pensions could increase the number of active nurses by 3.5%.[2]

Individual clinicians are capable of more and they know it. The OECD has compiled compelling evidence from doctors and nurses in many countries on the level of "skills mismatch" between what they have and what they need. Astonishingly, it found that 76% of doctors and 79% of nurses report performing tasks for which they are overqualified.[3]

However, the point here is not to argue that the effect of these policies might be to triple workforce capacity. Even if we wanted to, we could not maximize all policy levers simultaneously. Greece's long working hours, for example, are partly caused by low female participation in the economy, and in any case longer hours are often associated with, or even caused by, low productivity. The point is to demonstrate that demography is not destiny—government policies or national norms can significantly affect the healthcare workforce capacity.

End the cap?

At the other end of the generational scale, Generation Z—people born around 2000—are now making choices about their higher education and careers. Policy choices around the funding of higher education are at least as controversial as pension rights and benefits.

For decades, many OECD countries have regulated the number of clinical students admitted to universities and medical schools through quotas or *numerus clausus* policies, which limit student numbers. It is worth noting the sound arguments for this before moving the debate on. Quotas are often seen as barriers to entry to protect professional privileges, but there are reasons why they are so widespread. Hospitals have limited capacity to train large numbers of students to a high standard, while medical education is expensive and constrained by the public purse. Finally, some believe (especially for doctors) that numbers should be controlled to avoid oversupply, which could increase supply-induced demand. These reasons are sound but, in light of our impending global healthcare workforce shortage, I have reluctantly come to the conclusion that the benefits of this traditional approach no longer outweigh the drawbacks.

There are many more students trying to enter the caring professions than there are university places. The NHS currently employs about 26% of its doctors from abroad (often from poorer countries that cannot afford the brain drain) while large numbers of domestic applications to train are being turned down.[4] In 2018, there were close to 21,000 applicants for just over 6,500 places,[5] a potentially damaging neglect of talent. The year before, NHS spending on expensive agency staff to plug clinical vacancies was £1.3 billion[6]—the same as the amount spent on undergraduate medical training. While hospitals have now driven these agency staff costs down, the irony is that extra training posts, which reduce reliance on expensive locums, have been established outside normal training programmes. Where there is a will, there is always a way.

The UK's Royal College of Physicians has attempted a detailed analysis of future demand for doctors and the likely supply, looking at everything from medical school attrition rates to gender balance. They estimate that the total annual intake of medical students needs to be doubled over the next five years to about 15,000 if all branches of medicine are to have the staff they need by 2030.[7] This could well be a conservative estimate.

In Australia, the number of students admitted to nursing schools more than doubled between 2001 and 2013 from 8,000 to 19,000. Following the Bradley Review of 2008, the restrictive policies for entry into nursing education were abandoned. There is now a much healthier supply of nurses.[8]

Similarly, in the United Kingdom, pharmacy is now uncapped. In 2009 it was recognized as a 'shortage occupation', making overseas recruitment easier, but since then allowing universities to recruit according to student demand has eased the situation considerably, with few employers now reporting recruitment problems. The initiative has potentially overstimulated the supply, with the Centre for Workforce Intelligence estimating there could be between 11,000 and 19,000 surplus pharmacists by 2040.[9] However, this only compares supply with the demands of traditional pharmacy roles and not those needed across science, life sciences, and the growing number of occupational wellness programmes, to name just a few nontraditional opportunities. The United Kingdom has also opened up student places for physiotherapists—a profession, along with other allied health professionals, that is capable of doing much more if only it is allowed—leading to a jump of 15% between 2016 and 2017.

So should we supply more clinicians than are needed? While this is a rather basic way of posing the question, it strikes at the heart of the debate. In a paper for the Institute of Economic Affairs in 2017, Charlesworth and Lafond asked whether workforce planning needed a paradigm shift from undersupply to oversupply. They concluded that 'although an over-supply of some types of labour can add to cost pressures by increasing demand for health care services and … the cost of training is high, undersupply and poor labour planning lead to unintended consequences such as poor labour productivity. As a result there is a case for public policy to target an over-supply'.

I believe that in the face of enormous clinical and demographic challenges, we should press on with judicious deregulation of clinical supply for at least the next decade.

Professional regulation

As well as training more clinicians, governments should reform professional regulation; not to take aim at its noble purpose—that of assuring professional standards—but to reform slow, expensive, adversarial, and complex processes which act as a brake on innovative workforce practices.

To take one example, professional regulation needs to keep up with the pace of technological innovation and the resulting expansion in professional scopes of practice, but this rarely happens. In the United Kingdom, amendments to professional scopes of practice require a change in the law, a process that can take up to two years, or longer if challenged by other professional groups. Regulators should have the power to update regulation to reflect new working practices without constant recourse to legislation.

Professional regulation often impedes greater teamworking and integration of services. As scopes of practice expand and overlap, confusion can arise if the regulations governing teamworking are unclear. This is not helped by multiple regulatory bodies each operating separate rules of engagement. Professionals performing the same task may be regulated by separate bodies, each requiring a different burden of proof to demonstrate competence and each with a different disciplinary procedure for professionals found wanting. Under the circumstances, team members could be forgiven for being confused about each other's relative competence or their respective responsibilities.

Teamworking requires trust and understanding. Working without it leaves teams vulnerable to errors of omission or, where a culture of blame persists, to defensive work practices such as duplication or a disinclination to delegate. This is especially pertinent to 'virtual teams'—groups that are supposed to be integrated across the system but communicate by letter, referral, phone, and email rather than in person.

Regulation should facilitate the shift towards lifelong learning we need for our health professionals. Current education is heavily skewed towards pre-service training, despite the fact that much of what they learn ends up changing, as do the jobs they end up doing. Professional regulation of education standards could be a great lever to drive a more flexible, relevant, and up-to-date clinical workforce, if done in concert with other players such as universities.

There is also a need for the regulation of professionals to be more flexible across the career course. Rigid 'career escalators' that fast-track professionals to qualification can feel stifling for younger generations of clinicians. Many would prefer the opportunity to take time out—for family, research, innovation, or professional diversification. Younger professionals would also value being able to move across professions as they gain experience and skill. The new nursing associate role in the United Kingdom, for example, is a perfect gateway for healthcare assistants wanting to move into nursing later in their career.

As the Health Foundation has pointed out, who is 'in' and who is 'out' of statutory professional regulation is as much an accident of history as a rigorous, risk-based assessment.[10] Perfusionists, who operate heart and lung bypass machines during cardiac surgery, are unregulated. So are nursing assistants. Arts therapists, who use art to help people with emotional and behavioural issues, have been regulated in the United Kingdom for 15 years.

While there are several potential approaches to the problem, I can see merit in governments introducing a unifying piece of legislation covering all professional bodies. The UK's Professional Standards Authority for Health and Social Care—the regulators' regulator—is on the right lines in recommending a single, public-facing register of all health and care professionals with common professional standards[11] or at least a single code of practice. Fitness to practise cases involving more than one profession should be heard together, with an investigative and systems learning approach rather than an adversarial, punitive, and siloed one.

There is also widespread agreement about the need to focus more heavily on lifelong learning, and I would not be surprised if we eventually ended up regulating skills rather than roles. The neatest regulation I have seen is in Canada, where the whole of the nursing scope of practice consists of a brief statement about their common purpose and 14 controlled acts that qualified nurses can perform. The whole thing sits on a page of A4—now there's a challenge. The key information for each controlled act is spelt out in just a few words, covering issues such as prescribing, inserting instruments or fingers into the body, and managing the delivery of a baby. The Ontario document is a model of what good regulation should be— concise, proportionate, easily understood by both practitioners and the public, easily remembered, and directly relevant to the everyday work of the clinician.

Pay

Health is a caring, vocational practice, but even the most kind-hearted, altruistic, and empathic staff need to get decent pay. In addition, to have any chance of retaining them, it needs to keep up with pay in other sectors of the economy. The economic slowdown and subsequent austerity drives in the last decade left wages stalling across many OECD countries. But as the economy picked up in the private sector, public sector wages were left lagging (see Fig. 5.3). In the United Kingdom, the Health Foundation showed how nurses' wages started to fall behind everyone from garage managers and musicians to secretaries and crane drivers, going a long way to explaining falling entry rates and rising exits.

Those most likely to jump ship are on the lowest incomes and are early or late in their career, with less to lose. Hence the Deloitte finding that nurses were more inclined than doctors to leave, especially younger nurses and those close to retirement. The UK government was forced to remove the 1% pay cap on most health workers in 2018—two years earlier than planned—because of this effect.

Low public sector pay also leaves professions open to corruption and drives expansion in private provision. In China, corruption has eroded trust in public doctors so seriously that assaults are common.[12]

Finally, pay needs to keep pace with countries with whom you share mobility of labour. Europe is learning this lesson. The Slovak Republic, for instance, was forced to adopt a number of measures including pay increases to doctors and nurses to stop the exodus that occurred after accession to the European Union.

Earn, learn, and return

The current bias of governments towards the undersupply of clinical staff has created a global market for health professionals. Across the OECD, it is estimated that approximately 17% of all doctors and 6% of nurses are 'foreign-trained'. In countries

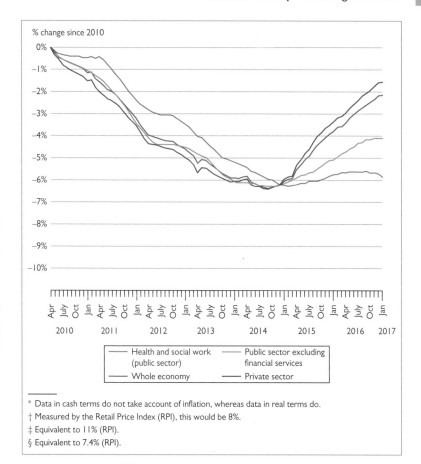

Fig. 5.3 Changes in pay since 2010, adjusted for consumer price index (CPI).

Reproduced with permission from Gershlick, B. et al. A sustainable workforce – the lifeblood of the NHS and social care. Election briefing May 2017. Copyright © The Health Foundation. Available at www.health.org.uk/publication/election-briefing-sustainable-workforce

such as the United States and United Kingdom, ranked first and second for the number of foreign-trained staff, the percentages are much higher. Destination countries like these have been criticised justifiably for benefitting from the investments of lower income countries that can ill afford the cost or loss. On the other hand, I can't help but reflect upon the fact that the history of humankind is the history of migration, with the global exchange of goods and services raising the prosperity and well-being of billions of people across the planet. As well as being a great way to spread outstanding clinical practice, international exchange promotes cultural diversity, helping nations to overcome prejudice and mistrust with tolerance and unity through a shared empathy in care.

For this reason, I echo the sentiments of the Global Code of Practice on the International Recruitment of Health Personnel, adopted by World Health Organization (WHO) member states in 2010 and supported by the Global Health Workforce Alliance. This guidance makes clear its expectations that countries should work towards being more self-sufficient in producing health staff, optimizing skill mix as well as increasing the overall stock of workers to improve performance, distribution, and productivity. In addition, however, the guidance gives tacit support to the ethical recruitment of health workers internationally through 'earn, learn, and return' schemes, a mutually beneficial approach I wholeheartedly support.

Heavy-handed attempts to cap student education numbers or reduce overseas-trained health professionals are regressive and short-sighted. A well-managed earn, learn, and return scheme coupled with open access to education helps individuals, international trade, and nation-building. It is the ultimate projection of soft power. The Mais Medicos programme, described in the Brazil chapter, was the perfect example of this approach.

Public health

The number of health workers required in 2030 will be profoundly affected by the way our health systems develop. Those that embrace health promotion and disease prevention could see significantly lower rates of ill health and a correspondingly reduced demand for services. Those that do not could face an accelerating and overwhelming surge.

As the most recent Global Burden of Disease Study has shown,[13] non-communicable diseases (NCDs) such as diabetes, heart disease, respiratory disease, and cancer are now the most significant drivers of health needs globally. The most insidious impact of these illnesses is not the deaths they cause but the increase in morbidity. While life expectancy has increased, broadly speaking, across the globe, the average number of disability-adjusted life years (DALYs) has increased, meaning people on average live longer lives but spend a greater portion of that life in ill health, dependent on health services and health personnel.

Unfortunately, while modern medicine has become adept at helping people live longer with chronic illness it has not yet made much of a dent in preventing it. This is the domain of public health, and public health is the domain of governments.

In 2011 the World Economic Forum published its list of 'best buy' public health interventions[14] to prevent NCDs that any government should be able to justify spending health dollars on. The list includes clinical interventions such as vaccinations and screening, but most of the measures are non-clinical. These include raising the price of alcohol, banning smoking in public places, and raising public awareness of the importance of good diet and physical activity. Some things only government can do.

Despite robust evidence, however, governments often overlook public health. Its funding is too easily ransacked for more prestigious projects or those with faster results, but few investments will deliver such benefits. As the only body with both the responsibility and the capacity to meet population health needs comprehensively, governments need to think long-term about public health to ensure the sustainability of their future health workforce.

Primary care-led health systems

As the disease burden shifts from acute short-term illness to chronic long-term care, so the focus of our health systems must shift from cure to care and from specialists to generalists. This could have profound implications for patient outcomes and work-force productivity. Integrated, population-based, primary health-led systems are far more efficient at managing the rising incidence of chronic illness and multimorbidity than siloed systems which reward fee for service activity. A US Medicare patient with one chronic condition typically sees four physicians per year, but this escalates to 14 physicians with five or more conditions. This is an incredibly inefficient use of human resources, which is why the WHO's health workforce strategy recommends that countries wanting to deliver universal health coverage pursue a primary health-led model.

Primary-led systems do not happen by accident. The optimal number of general-ists for this system is very different to the number generated under a system left to its own devices. For this reason, a degree of planning is required—usually but not necessarily by government.

Unfortunately, despite a need and desire for more generalists, general practice is declining in popularity across the globe. Between 2001 and 2010 there was a 6.3% decrease in the number of graduates entering primary care in the United States, but a 45% increase in those entering medical and surgical specialties. The United States predicts a 27% shortfall in adult generalist physicians by 2025.[15] In low- and middle-income countries, surveys of medical students showed a much higher preference for specialization over general practice, while in emerging markets such as Egypt, India, Jordan, Tunisia, and Turkey, fewer than 10% of physicians choose family medicine.

Expanding postgraduate training places for GPs is only part of the solution. Well-remunerated and attractive jobs must also be available on the other side. The OECD describes how GP wages have lagged specialty wages over the last 10–15 years, con-tributing to the suboptimal number of generalists. In low- and middle-income coun-tries, where private medical schools have flourished, regulation of training ratios may also be required. For countries lacking the fiscal or financial space to train more GPs and 'stuff their mouths with gold' as we did in the United Kingdom 15 years ago, 'mid-level providers' such as nurse practitioners in the United States or clinical officers in sub-Saharan Africa offer an alternative. Mid-level practitioners have the advantage of being as effective as primary care physicians at many things but taking less time and money to train and deploy—a feature which made them invaluable in scaling up the response to HIV/AIDS in sub-Saharan Africa.

Geographical distribution

All countries face issues with the regional distribution of staff. Left to market forces, doctors and nurses tend to live and work in the affluent urban areas and only governments face the unique responsibility of ensuring equitable access across landmass for their citizens. Governments generally have three options to address this problem: target current doctors, target future doctors, or cope with fewer doctors.[16]

Targeting current doctors is the carrot-and-stick approach and suits deprived urban areas more. The carrots are usually financial. Germany offers subsidies to GPs opening new practices in underserved areas, Canada offers bonuses for doctors in the most remote regions of British Columbia and in Alberta, financial incentives are used to help postpone retirement in rural areas. The sticks are most commonly regulatory. In Denmark, physician densities are capped through allocation of regional licences to practise and Germany has a similar system based on permits.

Targeting future doctors is an upstream measure. It means selecting and training staff in the places where they are needed most and works well in rural and remote regions. The Australian government subsidizes Bonded Medical Places that tie students in to a period of service in the most far-flung areas, Japan operates a regional quota system to ensure medical school places are distributed evenly across the prefectures, and the United Kingdom is expanding physician numbers by building medical schools in areas of need. The lead time on these policies is fairly long but there is good evidence now that marinating staff in the areas of need makes them more likely to stay in the long term—even better if they have come from there.

With such policies, it is important to take account of students' commitment to rural practice in the recruitment process, or graduates may leave after their bonded period of service. Medical schools are notorious for having the some of the highest-grade requirements for their courses but many would now argue that while those students are perfect for future careers in academic medicine, they may not be such good candidates for careers in rural and remote practice. Shifting the selection criteria requires cooperation between governments and training institutions, which often value the prestige of having such academically gifted recruits. This process is much easier I imagine when the institution is new—I hope so in the case of the new UK schools.

Finally, doing with fewer doctors means telemedicine, task shifting, and teamwork. Silver Chain, a healthcare provider in Australia, hosts holographic virtual clinics to ensure access to specialists for rural and remote patients and, of course, the Australians are well known for their flying doctors. France and Germany have piloted group practices in rural regions that take the strain off single-handed practitioners. In September 2018 French president Emmanuel Macron unveiled a series of measures including the redeployment of 400 doctors into rural areas and the creation of 4,000 extra roles, such that of doctors' assistants, to alleviate pressure. In Germany, family doctors are able to delegate home visits to trained non-physician practice assistants who do basic monitoring tasks such as blood pressure and glucose monitoring and routine medical care such as bandaging and injecting.

Overall, governments get a bad rap. Their rules and regulations conjure images of bureaucracy, red tape, and inertia. But when it comes to the role of the state, I prefer the more positive perspective of economist Mariana Mazzucato, author of *The Entrepreneurial State*. She argues that 'the state, far from being a hindrance to value creation, or an obstacle, has actually been the investor of first resort', and points out that many major technological advances from the internet to search algorithms and GPS have been stimulated by public investment.

Building partnerships

Governments exert extraordinary leverage over the health workforce nationally and internationally. They provide much of the funding, set standards and political priorities, have a huge impact on training and rewards, and determine the culture and rules for their national economy. Creative, agile, and sustained action by governments is central to tackling the global health workforce crisis.

Entrepreneurial governments will recognize they cannot solve the global or national workforce crisis on their own and they will create new partnerships, alliances, and joint ventures with community groups, charities, and industry. Officials will have to spend less time talking to themselves and more time building relationships outside highly demarcated and regimented institutional silos. The private sector will need to make sure it does not see the public sector as a series of sales targets, and instead view the relationship as an authentic commitment to mutual future prosperity. Nobody can solve this problem on their own.

Chapter 6

China—growth and social cohesion

I will never forget being in China during the reappointment of President Xi Jinping. Considered by many to be the most powerful Chinese leader since Mao Zedong, Beijing had more bunting than a British royal wedding. The Chinese people are looking to their leader to continue his drive to fight corruption and ensure economic growth is inextricably linked with social progress.

Big strides have been taken in universal healthcare, taking coverage from 45% in 2006 to over 97% today. While primary care is still uneven, this advance was only made possible with impressive developments that have a lineage from the barefoot doctors of the Communist revolution. Fast forward to 2019 and the Chinese government knows its health system will be unsustainable without a strong community network across this most populous country.

In the 20 years since I first visited China as part of an NHS delegation (to look for qualified nurses) the country has undergone a remarkable transformation into the global economic powerhouse we see growing before us today. The thousands of cyclists pedalling through the streets of Beijing in the early morning on their way to work gave way to vast numbers of cars, along with acrid smog. Therein lies the difficult balance the government is trying to strike between the benefits of economic progress and the adverse effects of such rapid urbanization and industrialization. The growth of the Chinese middle class, lifting so many from poverty, is enabled by the very same urbanization and industrialization that is affecting the physical and mental health of many.

From cancer to diabetes, obesity to cardiovascular disease, the chronic diseases of wealth are rising rapidly, while the health system is failing to keep up with people's soaring demand for quality healthcare. But it should not be forgotten how far China has already come—implementing the world's largest basic healthcare coverage. The question is whether it can pick up the pace in terms of the reach and depth of care provision, with many patients still incurring significant out of pocket expenses.

The Chinese need to improve access to healthcare and its quality at a speed and scale that almost defies comprehension, in a country where six of the 33 provincial administrations have populations greater than France, and three are larger than one million square kilometres. The healthcare industry is expected to become a US$1 trillion a year business by 2020, with one of the highest annual growth rates globally. This covers a population of 1.4 billion people served by 3.8 million registered nurses, 3.4 million licensed doctors, and over 31,000 hospitals. While the numbers are astonishing, they are still relatively low by global standards. China has 2.4 doctors for every 1,000 people, with a plan to raise this to 2.5 by 2020.[1] The Organisation for Economic Co-operation and Development (OECD) average is

3.4.[2] Similarly, the low number of nurses at 2.7 per 1,000 in 2017 should increase to 3.1 by 2020. Only around 1% of registered nurses are male, largely due to the effect of traditional gender stereotypes.[3] Countering this may help address some of the shortfalls.

The distribution of the healthcare workforce across such a vast country is also a problem, with too many gravitating to big cities. Beijing alone accounts for roughly a fifth of healthcare spending. Only 15% of doctors working in primary care, and around 90% of healthcare interactions take place in hospital compared with around 10% in the United Kingdom. For these reasons primary care is frequently cited as the weakest link in Chinese healthcare.

The government is well aware of these shortcomings. Healthcare is now central to China's plans for development, attempting to balance economic growth with the desire for a higher quality of life, particularly among the growing middle classes. Xi Jinping and Premier Li Keqiang have called for faster improvements in primary care. In his marathon address to the 19th Party Congress in 2017, President Xi identified a healthy population as a mark of a prosperous and strong country. In pursuit of the Healthy China reform drive, he promised a wide range of measures including improvements to primary care, more GPs, better hospital management, an end to the practice of hospitals funding their operations with profits from overpriced drugs and support for the development of private hospitals. The framework for the Healthy China 2030 Plan has the number of registered doctors as a core indicator. Achieving the government's goals will depend on delivering their pledge to improve the status of an overworked and underpaid health workforce, especially primary care providers, to improve recruitment and retention. One significant cultural step towards this has been the 'special glory' of a new 'Medical Workers Day' on 19 August every year, initiated by health authorities and the government to call for respect from society for the nation's health workers.[4]

Without growing a primary care system, it is difficult to see how China will cope with rising demand, but the scale of this challenge is immense. According to the National Health and Family Planning Commission (now replaced by the National Health Commission), China needs to train more than 150,000 general practitioners by 2020.[5] It has looked overseas for help with this huge effort. Among other collaborations, a partnership with Health Education England, the University of Nottingham Ningbo Campus and Ningbo First Hospital is examining how China can strengthen its primary care training, and University of Birmingham is working with Sun-Yat Sen University in Guangdong province to develop a primary care training centre.

These huge shortfalls extend to other specialty areas, with an estimated 140,000 new obstetricians, 90,000 paediatricians and 40,000 psychiatrists required.[6,7,8] Supplying these will be a monumental task, not helped by the poor employment conditions in the health service.

The case for dramatic expansion is made more urgent by the rapidly ageing population (Fig. 6.1). The now rescinded one-child policy has exacerbated this, with relatively low birth rates reducing the working-age workforce available in the years ahead, the impact of which will take several generations to change. As the demographic of the country shifts to an older society, the need for more healthcare workers will grow.

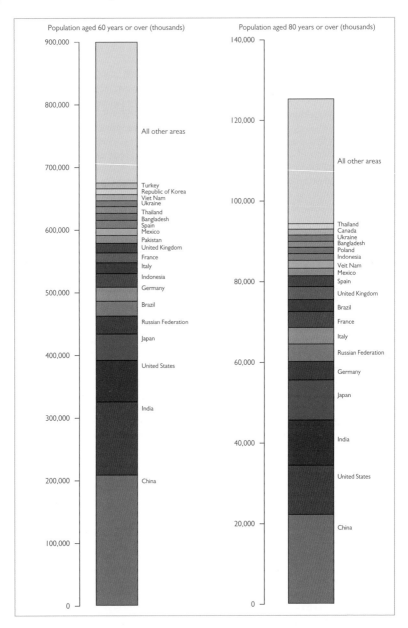

Fig. 6.1 Population ages 60 years or over and aged 80 years or over by country, 2015.

Source: data from United Nations, Department of Economic and Social Affairs, Population Division (2015). World Population Prospects: The 2015 Revision, Key Findings and Advance Tables. Working Paper No. ESA/P/WP.241. Copyright © 2015 United Nations.

Low pay, high pressure, and violence

Going to the doctor has long been a headache for the Chinese, and the public sector system is under huge pressure. In the absence of a comprehensive primary care system, patients flock to top hospitals, often queuing for hours for just a couple of minutes with a physician.

These design flaws, and patients' preference to be seen by doctors at the main public hospitals, are exacerbated by the shortage of healthcare staff to see them. This contributes to patient and family frustration, with medical staff reporting high levels of aggression. Violent attacks and even murders have been common. Laws introduced in 2015 to protect staff have led to at least 8,000 people being prosecuted for intentionally injuring someone or inciting crowds at hospitals, and there are indications that this is helping get the problem under control.[9] Great efforts to manage patient and family expectations, protect staff, and stop violence are required to encourage people back into the healthcare workforce.

Low pay is a long-standing cause of many problems. Doctors in the public system are typically paid in the region of US$22,000–29,000, supplemented by payments and other benefits from pharmaceutical and medical device companies. This kickback culture has been widely criticised, and the government has tried to take action. Medical graduates are increasingly voting with their feet by choosing other professions or going abroad.

But despite its shortcomings, doctors largely prefer roles in public sector institutions over better-paid private providers. Several factors contribute to this. Though slowly changing, the public's perception is that private providers (outside the top providers, usually backed by international money) generally deliver lower levels of care. Research and teaching facilities within state providers are a source of prestige, and this, coupled with job stability, mean that the private healthcare sector struggles to attract physicians. This is despite a rule change in 2017 that allows multipractice working, designed to help develop the private sector and take some pressure off the public system. Unfortunately, permission is often required from the base employer, and given staff shortages, many public hospitals do not want to let their doctors go. In Beijing, just 4% of physicians work in multiple clinics.[10]

Valuing nurses

Nursing is a particularly undervalued and underprivileged job, with low pay, poor working conditions, and high workloads. Nursing was only re-established as a post-schooling discipline in China in 1983. Levels of responsibility are low compared with many other countries and there is little opportunity for skill development or career progression. Given this, the huge undersupply of nurses should come as little surprise, but it is exacerbated by high levels of often unpaid overtime, unpredictable shifts, and wide variations in pay and conditions.

While there are trade unions, they are likely to be controlled by management and act as a bridge between the Communist Party and the staff. There is an urgent need for greater staff support to ensure they feel listened to and valued.

Recent government reforms outline an increased role for nursing, with wider clinical responsibilities, but there are concerns that a rapid expansion in numbers risks diluting the quality of training. Traditionally fulfilling a more subservient role in healthcare, the scope for allowing nursing to advance up to and beyond the level of responsibility seen in other healthcare systems offers a significant opportunity to address healthcare shortcomings.

The Sanming experiment

One of the most fascinating Chinese examples of redesigning a healthcare system is the city of Sanming.[11] I have visited this health system on several occasions and have great respect for its successes and ambitions. Like the rest of China's public hospital sector, it has faced numerous problems including under-the-counter payments to doctors, inefficiency, and serious financial pressures. In 2012 it began to implement a reform package which has since become a national pilot scheme being followed by other cities.

Drug mark-ups by hospitals were banned and reforms to drug financial controls streamlined drug supply chains, slashed fraud, and exposed poor performance. Combined with centralized procurement, substantial savings were generated (see Fig. 6.2) which were reinvested in the doubling of salaries, more generous insurance benefits, and a centralized management structure that could keep much tighter control. Hospital chief executives were given proper annual salary packages and subjected to a comprehensive performance management system based on the quality of care and operations. The huge salary increases meant doctors no longer felt in the pocket of drug companies, leading to tangible improvements in staff satisfaction and motivation. Most staff are now happy with their income—a rare achievement in Chinese healthcare.

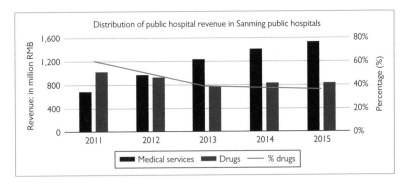

Fig. 6.2 Distribution of public hospital revenue in Sanming public hospitals.

Technological leaps

Much has been written about the rapid technological development of China, set as a strategic priority by the government and often facilitated by close working links with the country's own tech giants. The fragmented, government-run public health system has been slow to digitize, so the drive for this is being led by the private sector. China is pouring investment into research and development across the board, and Premier Li Keqiang has said that healthcare tech could 'help alleviate the problem of inaccessible and expensive public health services that have long been a big concern'.[12]

The scale of this digital innovation, driven by necessity and ambition, means China could use technology to bridge some of the workforce gap much faster than training up new staff. An example is the WeDoctor mobile health platform, backed by Chinese multinational Tencent, offering online consultations and doctor appointments. It has over 160 million registered customers and a company valuation of US$5.5 billion.[13] Similarly, Ping An Good Doctor, backed by Ping An Insurance, uses its online health platform to connect users with a nationwide network of healthcare service providers covering 3,100 hospitals, 1,100 health check-up centres, 500 dental clinics, and 7,500 pharmacies.[14] The service has grown to over 190 million registered users in just four years. Many health systems can learn from this approach.

China is racing to develop artificial intelligence (AI) tools in many areas, and healthcare is a major target with over 130 companies already applying AI to areas such as automating routine medical tasks.[15] Here, China has the advantage of scale. With such a large population the healthcare data that is the source of AI algorithms is vast, restrictions around its use are less stringent than in many Western countries, and there is little public awareness of the issues around privacy and data security.

One widely reported example is the Guangzhou Second Provincial Hospital, which is working with several private companies to deploy this technology. Based on over 300 million medical records, an AI tool has been trained to provide prediagnosis with a claimed accuracy of more than 90% for over 200 diseases,[16] helping patients to seek support from the most appropriate physician.

Other potential applications are myriad. Chinese tech giant Alibaba is working with a Shanghai hospital to predict patient demand and allocate doctors, while in Zhejiang the company is developing AI-assisted diagnosis tools to help automate reading of computed tomography (CT) and magnetic resonance imaging (MRI) scans.[17] Meanwhile, the Chinese company iFlytek has developed an AI doctor assistant to listen to doctors with patients and produce e-documents for patient reports, even suggesting prescriptions, to help save doctors time. Their medical robot famously passed China's medical licence examination in 2017, becoming the world's first robot to pass such a test.[18]

Intriguingly, an MIT technology review highlights different perceptions about the impact of AI on medicine in China and the West. While Western doctors debate fears about job losses, Chinese doctors appear keener to automate the most repetitive tasks.[19]

While the speed of digital development in China is impressive, it needs to be balanced with greater regulatory oversight; otherwise technological advances will outrun the understanding of the impact on safety and ethics.

Conclusion

China's serious problem with under-the-counter payments to doctors is an extreme example of what can happen when a healthcare workforce is undervalued. The pernicious problem of violence towards healthcare staff can only add to the feeling that their expertise and contribution are poorly recognized and rewarded.

But the Sanming example shows what can be achieved in just a few years with determined leadership with the courage to address the root causes of deep-seated difficulties. While it has required significant investment of money and resources, it has slashed the corrosive effects of dishonesty, raised morale, and freed clinical staff to do the job they always wanted to do. Key to this success has been the brave fight against corruption, alongside transparency and higher pay, which has helped incentivize the right behaviours in the system. This is far more effective than simply trying to root out 'a few bad apples'. For patients, it has delivered more healthcare at higher quality. Sanming shows the path that Chinese healthcare needs to take.

Finally, there is a global race for supremacy in AI and China, like America, is investing tremendous resources and power into this area for a wide variety of sectors, including defence, smart cities, and healthcare. It would not surprise me if some of the quickest innovations and adaptations in health AI come from the East. It is needed domestically and will be exported globally.

Chapter 7

Patients as partners and communities as carers—renewable energy

Healthcare systems are slowly grasping the revolutionary potential of empowering patients to play a more active role in their own care. But making this a reality requires overhauling the nature of the relationship between patients and staff and re-skilling both the staff and the patients.

Healthcare is more than a decade behind industries such as retail and banking in developing their customers' capacity to create value. In healthcare, payers and clinicians are starting to realize the opportunities for harnessing patient power to drive quality, improve lifestyles, and control costs (see Fig. 7.1), with a particular focus on managing the growing burden of chronic diseases, while patient groups are demanding more power over their own care.

Many organizations think they are empowering patients already; patients overwhelmingly say they are not. Healthcare has been slow to exploit this potential in part because it has traditionally been viewed as a moral rather than an economic issue—the right thing to do rather than crucial to making healthcare systems sustainable. Patient power is also a difficult concept for medicine because it changes the relationship between clinicians and patients.

To be truly transformative, enabling patients to be partners in their own care means rethinking every step of the healthcare process, from how research is conducted to how services are designed, the offer made to patients, how decisions are taken, and how outcomes are judged. The alignment between what patients want and what is provided is often poor. The goals of patients are not given enough recognition in treatment choices, and the benefits of shared decision-making and patient and carer involvement are not being realized. The result is that in many parts of the world overdiagnosis and overtreatment are a frequent hazard and serious cost.

Patient power reflects core healthcare values of dignity, respect, and safety and recognizes the particular needs and aspirations of each patient, carer, and community. It also drives efficiency by improving the outcomes that matter to patients and stimulating the development of new models of care. But delivering it requires the entire system to be directed towards creating high-quality outcomes and experiences for patients. This in turn requires a culture of continuous improvement and a decisive move away from setting goals around the work of individual teams or departments rather than the overall value created for the patient's journey.

Dr Albert Mulley, director of the Dartmouth Center for Health Care Delivery Science in the United States, believes there is a widespread failure by clinicians to

Patient activation

Many studies have shown that patients who are activated — i.e. have the skills, ability, and willingness to manage their own health and healthcare — have better health outcomes at lower costs compared with less activated patients. Judith Hibbard of the University of Oregon has developed a 'patient activation measure'— a validated survey that scores the degree to which patients see themselves as a manager of their health and care.

Patients with the lowest activation scores, that is, people with the least skills and confidence to actively engage in their own healthcare, cost 8–21% more than patients with the highest activation levels, even after adjusting for health status and other factors. And patient activation scores were shown to be significant predictors of healthcare costs.[5]

Predicted per capita costs of patients by patient activation level

2010 patient activation level	Predicted per capita billed costs (US$)	Ratio of predicted costs relative to level 4 Patient Activation Measure (PAM)
Level 1 (lowest)	966	1.21
Level 2	840	1.05
Level 3	783	0.97
Level 4 (highest)	799	1.00

Fig. 7.1 Patient activation.

Reproduced with permission from Creating new value with patients, carers and communities.

understand their patients' preferences and how proposed interventions will affect their lives. This 'preference misdiagnosis' wastes resources and can harm patients. There is also growing concern about overdiagnosis, in which patients are overinvestigated and screened, and sometimes harmed as a result.

A patient who is fully informed of their treatment options and risks will often make decisions about their care which are more conservative and lower cost than the course recommended by their physician. This means they are more likely to get an outcome with which they are happy while saving the system money.

Shared decision-making involves developing skills to help patients understand their condition and treatment options and to express their preferences. This means training staff, developing health coaches to work alongside the patient, providing decision aids and documenting and tracking preferences. One of the barriers to this approach is that many clinicians support the principle but feel they do not have the time. Like many healthcare reforms it requires investment—putting in the time and effort upfront to involve the patient in order to secure a more satisfactory outcome for them while saving resources overall.

According to Nesta—the United Kingdom's innovation foundation—involving patients, their families, and communities more directly in the management of long-term health conditions could save the NHS £4.4 billion, through cuts in emergency hospital admissions, planned admissions, and outpatient appointments.[1] Numerous studies suggest the cost of managing patients with long-term conditions could be reduced by up to 20%. Nesta estimates the annual cost of what it calls People Powered Health at between £100 and £400 per patient. But savings of this magnitude can only be realized if healthcare systems make the shift from high cost, unplanned, hospital-based care models to more effective co-management of conditions in the community.

Shifting the power

Patient empowerment needs to be hardwired into training and development, to drive a shift from the paternalistic and overwhelmingly medical culture which dominates healthcare to one which embraces patients as partners and gives far greater recognition to the social determinants of health.

While training is still largely focused on the treatment of episodic illnesses, clinicians need the skills to help patients manage their own conditions and behaviours over months and years and be partners in decisions about their care. This requires excellent communication skills, empathy, collaboration with the patient and colleagues, negotiation, shared decision-making, and problem-solving.[2]

But as the UK's Institute for Public Policy Research notes, achieving these changes will be a profound challenge. It means confronting a mindset honed and embedded over centuries of medical practice.[3] It calls into question the very basis of the doctor/patient relationship, where the power of the physician comes from their monopoly of knowledge and ability to determine treatment.

Doctors will need to get to grips with tools which guide them through the techniques of shared decision-making, and be trained in building a care plan around the patient's wider objectives rather than focusing almost exclusively on clinical aims.[4] This means accepting that they are one part of a productive partnership rather than the expert in every aspect of the care plan.

Implementing and maintaining this patient-centred approach will require intense and sustained leadership at all levels of the healthcare system, embedding the new ethos in the values of every organization and in the practicalities of every care pathway. It is no less than a social reordering of healthcare, with the old hierarchy being replaced with a more equal relationship between doctor and patient. This is simple to describe but hard to deliver.

Giving patients the tools

At least as difficult will be providing the support to patients to enable them to make the most of this new relationship. This in turn will depend on training people such as GPs, practice nurses, care navigators, volunteers, and peers in how to pass on the skills.

Non-clinical staff and volunteers will be crucial to the success of any moves towards greater patient empowerment. They will help patients develop the tools, techniques, and understanding of how to make the most of this new relationship as well as keeping their side of the bargain by striving to achieve shared goals such as making lifestyle changes.[5] While the majority of this chapter is dedicated to patients and carers, it is worth acknowledging the crucial role volunteers play. A recent King's Fund report for the United Kingdom suggested there were around three million people volunteering in health and social care, making a vital contribution to patient, carer, staff, and visitors' experience.

But training both patients and staff is difficult. Training patients does not fit the way health services are delivered in most developed countries, while it is hard to engage time-poor clinicians in the practicalities of making this new relationship work. An evaluation of an expert patient programme in the United Kingdom concluded that community-based training in self-care 'is not yet accepted as a core part of long-term condition management within health professional cultures. It was a concept that was divorced from the concrete reality of dealing with patients in everyday clinical practice'.[6]

It will take more than a couple of afternoons and some flipcharts to overhaul a professional lifetime of ingrained culture. Sporadic training programmes have virtually no hope of securing change. The only way to make it stick is to have it ingrained in the way people think and work from their first day of instruction, alongside a massive training, support, and communication programme aimed at existing staff and system leaders.

On the patient side, training depends on building a volunteer workforce of people who have practical experience as expert patients. Finding people who are likely to make good trainers and who can commit considerable time to the programme, and then ensuring a reasonable consistency in how the training is delivered, is difficult and time-consuming.

For mental health in particular, the workforce needs to meet the needs of families as well as patients. In Birmingham, the Meridien Family Programme run by Birmingham and Solihull Mental Health NHS Foundation Trust trains staff to provide more family-sensitive mental health services, with a focus on involving the families in supporting the patient, as well as helping the entire family in problem solving and stress management.[7]

In the United Kingdom, avoidable emergency admissions are placing a severe strain on the entire healthcare system. Among the many interventions to try to get a grip on this problem, Vale of York Clinical Commissioning Group set up a trial with York Teaching Hospital NHS Foundation Trust and Swedish company Health Navigator to provide telephone support for patients who were at high risk of emergency admissions. The aims were to help patients look after themselves better, and to understand the care options available to them when they needed help, so they would not simply turn up at the emergency department. Weekly coaching calls in the randomized trial resulted in 63% fewer non-elective admissions, 60% fewer A&E attendances, and 17% fewer bed days. In terms of costs, the project was close to breaking even in its first year.[8]

This simple and highly effective project shows how giving staff the skills to communicate with patients in new ways can deliver significant success in improving patients' quality of life and reducing pressure on the system.

Patient involvement can be used to understand how they perceive different parts of a service and the value they receive. In particular, talking to patients helps identify steps that should be removed, improving the patient experience while driving up productivity. There are many ways of using the experiences of patients and carers in service design, such as interviews, observations, diaries, stories, and ethnography.

Involving patients in service design is a different way of thinking about teams, organizations, structures, flows, productivity, and outcomes. Analysing the system through the eyes of the patient will challenge clinical hierarchies, question the value of different skills, and overturn long-established patterns of behaviour. It is difficult work which takes time to get right, but it can have a profound effect on patient experience, care quality, and system efficiency.

A few tasks can even be shifted from staff to patients in hospital. While most of us are used to self-service check-in for airports, it is an approach that has only been tried rarely in hospitals. However, self-service check-ins when arriving for outpatient appointments and routine operations would save money by streamlining administrative tasks, automating systems, reducing errors, and making arrival quicker and easier for patients.[9]

A hospital in Mysore, India has taken the self-service idea even further by involving family members in providing postoperative care. Working with Stanford University in the United States, the Narayana Health hospital has developed a four-hour audio and video curriculum explaining how to care for patients during the three-day recovery period following heart surgery. This helps ensure continuity of care at home and reduces postsurgical complications. While there are obviously risks with taking the role of carer to this extreme, it is nonetheless a striking example of how healthcare systems in developing countries which are unable to pursue traditional care models can squeeze every last piece of value out of the resources they have available. It is not that far removed from family members looking after patients when they return home from day surgery.

Empowering patients through apps and wearables

Apps and wearables are driving increasing numbers of citizens to feel a sense of responsibility for, and control over, their health and well-being, by checking, tracking, and transmitting health metrics. Information that can be collected and analysed ranges from respiratory rate, hydration, and blood glucose to ECG traces, autonomic nervous activity, sleep patterns, and stress levels.

A study by Imperial College Health Partners in London of three apps to help patients manage Type 2 diabetes shows the extraordinary potential for people to take control of long-term conditions. Between 53% and 80% of participants completed an app-based programme, compared with less than 7% for face-to-face programmes.[10]

The most effective apps take a 'whole life' approach, integrating medical records and diagnostics with comprehensive, evidence-based information supporting both physical and mental health.

One of the biggest barriers to mobilizing the power of apps is poor understanding among clinicians of what is available and how users can gain the most benefit. A study by the West Midlands Academic Health Science Network in the United Kingdom found that poor understanding among doctors, nurses, and service commissioners of what technology can offer patients was holding back adoption. DigitalHealth. London quoted a survey in the United States by Medscape exposing sharp differences between doctors and patients about whether patients should be empowered to use technology. While 39% of patients said they would like to use smartphone apps to self-diagnose non-life-threatening medical conditions, only 18% of physicians agreed. Only 58% of physicians agreed with the statement 'new technology must be mastered to remain up-to-date'.[11]

The hidden army of carers

In the Mysore example, the family members are engaged in significant caring for just a few days. But family members—often the women—can be caught up in providing care for months or years, typically for the frail elderly but also for children with significant disabilities who might not have survived in previous generations. In all but name, these carers become part of the healthcare workforce.

The size of this near-invisible workforce is astonishing. Across the OECD, more than one in 10 adults is involved in informal, typically unpaid, caregiving.[12] There is no clear pattern. For example, some southern European countries such as Italy and Spain have among the highest percentages, but nearby Greece ranks among the lowest, alongside Denmark and Sweden, where there are high levels of state support. While carers are obviously primarily concerned with looking after close relatives, almost one in five help a friend or neighbour.

Developing the right role for carers is a difficult and sensitive issue. There is a fine balance between providing more support for carers and dumping significant responsibilities on them. High-intensity caring—taken as at least 20 hours per week—tends to reduce people's ability to hold down a full-time job, so it can be associated with poverty. It can also be stressful and socially restricting—you can't get out of the house. This, particularly where it is associated with a lack of support, can in turn lead to mental health problems for the carer. The OECD estimates that the prevalence of mental health conditions among carers is a fifth higher than among non-carers. So apart from the obvious human cost, unsupported caring can create its own demand for healthcare.[13]

A large number of OECD countries encourage and support caring through financial incentives, either paid directly to carers or to those receiving the care. Countries such as Canada and the United States offer tax credits, while in Finland, municipal authorities pay family caregivers directly at a fairly generous rate. English-speaking countries such as Australia, Ireland, New Zealand, and the United Kingdom have means-tested benefits.

Systems attempting to channel cash to carers are inevitably complex, trading off factors such as the intensity of care provided, the time it takes, the relationship between the carer and the person being cared for, other income and the impact it has on their employment opportunities.

Increasingly, there is a tendency to channel cash through the care recipient. This is seen as encouraging the independence of the person needing care, as well as empowering them to shape how their care is provided. As the OECD study recognizes, providing support in this way has the advantage of simpler eligibility criteria directly linked to the needs of the individual. The downside is that it can monetize family relationships.

In 1995, Germany introduced Long Term Care Insurance (LTCI). Participation was mandatory and the insurance would pay out if patients required care for six months or longer. It was explicitly for care and excluded what they refer to as 'hotel' costs— this becomes particularly relevant when beneficiaries move into residential care as they can still face high out of pocket payments.

The purpose of LTCI was not to offer comprehensive state protection, but to change expectations about the role of family and friends in providing care. They were expected to be the primary carers, while the state would help those families keep their loved ones at home for longer. Sometimes this was services in kind, sometimes it was cash payments, and sometimes a mixture. The cash payments were popular, with two-thirds going for that option (15% chose a mix of both), despite the fact that cash payments were only half the monetary value of services in kind.

The number of beneficiaries requiring formal care from state providers dropped sharply. But this did not mean the need for them fell away—around this time the number of care workers from Central and Eastern Europe started to rise. Some were formally employed, others illegally. Many were employed as residential 24-hour carers for beneficiaries with dementia or other high care needs. It is estimated between 150,000 and 200,000 migrant carers came this way.

Some countries are against the idea of care allowances. Japan, which has similar long-term care insurance, rejected the cash payments option. Women's lobbying groups opposed it, arguing that help was needed rather than cash; with limited access to migrant labour and an already tight labour market, cash payments would simply formalize traditional caring roles for women, and hold back ambitions to raise the female participation rate in the shrinking workforce.

Community power

As well as tapping into the resources of patients and groups, some healthcare systems are mobilizing the resources of entire communities to deliver culturally appropriate services at low cost. It is not easy—cultural sensitivity is vital and community engagement is paramount—but the potential is huge.

Implicit in this approach is that healthcare organizations and staff cede power to those communities. An impressive example is the Nuka System of Care provided for over 30 years by the Southcentral Foundation in Anchorage, Alaska, and driven by the Alaska Native people. It is infused with the culture of this region, which recognizes that disease and its treatment has social, psychological, and cultural components as well medical. The patient is treated as a customer and owner of their care system; treatment is founded on long-term relationships with teams that understand each person's values, goals, priorities, and strengths and provides an integrated approach to the mind, body, and spirit alongside a commitment to measurement and quality. Since its inception, Nuka has secured a 50% reduction in emergency room and urgent care visits, striking results for illness prevention and screening and a cultural respect rating of 99.2%.[14]

Countries such as Bangladesh, India, Malawi, and Nepal are using women's groups to try to reduce deaths during pregnancy and childbirth.[15] Around 270,000 women die every year from pregnancy and childbirth complications, while around three million infants do not survive their first month. The groups identify and prioritize health problems around childbirth and develop local strategies to overcome them. Role-playing and storytelling are among the techniques used to boost women's confidence to talk about these issues and to change their own and others' behaviour.

Seismic change

The advantages to both patients and healthcare systems of making citizens partners in their care are obvious, but the barriers to making it happen are immense. It needs nothing less than overhauling a medical culture developed over centuries which says the doctor knows best. I don't know a health system in the world that will be sustainable without patients taking greater responsibility for their care. It's no longer a nicety, it's a necessity.

Chapter 8

The Netherlands—zorg in de gemeenschap

I admire the Dutch for their disdain of insincerity and hypocrisy. Their proud history of being an adventurous, bold (some might say blunt) seafaring people trading across the world has given them a wonderful open culture that blends entrepreneurship with social solidarity. This is reflected in their health and aged care system, considered by some to be one of the finest in the world because of its pioneering provision and decent level of funding. 'Zorg in de gemeenschap' or 'care in the community' is a both a distinguishing and defining feature of the Dutch cure and care system.

The Dutch spend around 3.7% of their gross domestic product (GDP) on long-term care,[1] the highest in the Organisation for Economic Co-operation and Development (OECD), and offer many examples of innovation in caring for older people in the community and at home. Nearly 13% of the population aged over 65 receive care at home, compared with just 4.9% across the OECD.[2]

Primary care first

A strength of the Dutch healthcare system is the emphasis placed on well-resourced primary care. The Dutch government supports GPs because it sees them as allies in controlling the cost of secondary care. With such a huge proportion of the economy already dedicated to healthcare, Dutch politicians are acutely aware that they cannot spend their way out of trouble, so controlling cost pressures is a big and growing problem.

In recent years there has been rapid consolidation in primary care, with GPs increasingly working in larger settings such as healthcare centres supported by allied healthcare staff and managers. Growing numbers of GPs see themselves as part of a multidisciplinary team rather than a stand-alone doctor.[3] A lot of community pharmacists formally collaborate with local GPs (although the Netherlands has far fewer pharmacists for its size than many European countries; Belgium has six times as many per 100,000 population).

This integrated, collaborative approach is encouraging new ways of working and new types of worker, including practice nurses, nurse practitioners, nurse specialists, and physician assistants. This willingness to embrace change and learn new skills chimes with the findings of a PwC survey of 11 countries, which found that the Dutch

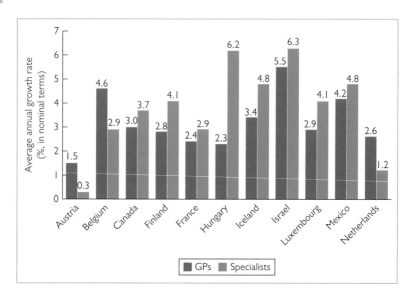

Fig. 8.1 Growth in the remuneration of GPs and specialists, 2005–2013 (or nearest year).
Reproduced with permission from Buchan, J. et al. (Eds). Health Employment and Economic Growth: An Evidence Base. Geneva, Switzerland: World Health Organization. Copyright © 2017 WHO.

workforce was by far the most adaptable, significantly ahead of countries such as the United Kingdom, Singapore, and the United States.[4]

General practice is the most popular specialization for medical students, followed by paediatrics, internal medicine, and surgery.[5] Around a fifth of medical graduates eventually become GPs. The Netherlands in one of just a few countries where general practitioner pay has grown faster than that of specialists (see Fig. 8.1), putting primary care in a strong position to attract talent.

GPs are a powerful voice in the system. The National Association of General Practitioners negotiates over issues such as salaries and how general practice is organized, while the Dutch College of General Practitioners publishes its own guidelines on the treatment of around a hundred conditions in primary care.[6] This means guidelines are crafted by GPs specifically for primary care rather than being handed down by some remote national body. All this helps raise the prestige and profile of general practice.

The combination of better facilities, better support, and better collaboration makes being a GP a highly attractive option for medical graduates, and contrasts strongly with the United Kingdom, where the talk is of burnout, crisis, unfilled posts, underfunding, closing surgeries, and early retirement. In 2017, 1,250 graduates competed for 750 trainee posts, while in the United Kingdom 451 trainee posts were left unfilled.[7] There is also anecdotal evidence that medical students in the Netherlands are given a more positive impression of general practice.

The Buurtzorg phenomenon

For some, the Dutch health system is synonymous with the Buurtzorg community nursing care company. Of course, it's not, but its innovative structure cuts bureaucracy and gives nurses more freedom and time with clients. It deploys self-governing teams of up to 12 nurses who are responsible for between 40 and 60 people within a particular area. Each nurse is capable of meeting the full range of the patient's needs from medical requirements to support services, which had traditionally been provided by cheaper, less highly trained staff. There are now around 900 teams in the Netherlands caring for tens of thousands of patients, supported by just a few dozen administrators and trainers.

The principle underpinning the model is that the nurse acts as a health coach for the individual and their family, emphasizing preventive health measures and maximizing their independence through self-care, supported by networks of neighbourhood resources. The massive national and international publicity that Buurtzorg has generated has helped it attract talented staff, and its workforce satisfaction levels are as impressive as those of the clients.

In 2015 the health ministry commissioned KPMG in the Netherlands to analyse Buurtzorg's performance. We found that they were indeed a lower cost provider of good quality home-care services (scoring strikingly high net promoter and employee satisfaction scores) and—contrary to claims by some of its critics—this was not because they were cherry-picking patients. Compared with the average home-care organization, Buurtzorg patients were more likely to go into nursing homes at a younger age but subsequent care costs were lower (probably due to relative better health when they went into a nursing home). When the patients' nursing home and hospital costs were added in, the total cost per patient was about average for the Netherlands (see Fig. 8.2).[8] Buurtzorg has had a powerful effect on the homecare industry, with some of its competitors adopting similar ways of working.

Planning ahead

The Netherlands has a sophisticated system for planning its medical workforce. Attempting to allocate healthcare staff efficiently is an economic necessity, with health and care services accounting for well over 16% of the Dutch workforce—a total which has grown by about a fifth since the early 2000s—and around 10.1% of GDP.[9] It is a hybrid Bismarckian social insurance system.

For many years, the Netherlands has used a demand-led forecasting model to enable centralized decision-making about the appropriate number of medical and specialist training places for doctors, aiming to avoid either shortages or oversupply (preventing supply-induced demand through training too many staff is an important objective). The system was established after a looming shortage of GPs and medical specialists became apparent in the late 1990s.

The model looks around 15–20 years ahead, and is inevitably an imperfect science. Elements it attempts to assess include labour market migration, sociocultural developments, changes in working hours, technical developments, efficiency changes, and the movement of tasks within and between professions.[10]

	Buurtzorg	Other Dutch home-care providers
Average hours of home care (per client per year)	108 hours	168 hours
Average home-care costs (excluding follow-up costs)	€6,428 ($6,990)	€7,995 ($8,695)
Average follow-up costs in the Exceptional Medical Expense Act (mainly nursing home cost)	€2,029 ($2,207)	€2,510 ($2,730)
Average follow-up medical (physician and hospital) costs	€7,787 ($8,468)	€5,187 ($5,641)
Total case-mix adjusted cost per client, (Including home care and follow-up costs)	€15,357' ($16,701)	€15,856* ($17,243)

* Only the total costs include ease-mix adjustment.

Source: KPMG, *The Added Value of Buurtzorg Relative to Other Providers of Home Care: A Quantitative Analysis of Home Care in the Netherlands in 2013* [in Dutch], Jan. 2015.

Fig. 8.2 Cost comparison: Buurtzorg vs. other Dutch home-care providers.

Reproduced with permission from KPMG. (2015) The Added Value of Buurtzorg Relative to Other Providers of Home Care: A Quantitative Analysis of Home Care in the Netherlands in 2013 [in Dutch] / KPMG-Plexus. De toegevoegde waarde van Buurtzorg t.o.v. andere aanbieders van thuiszorg. Eeen kwantiatieve analyse van thuiszorg in Nederland anno 2013. Copyright 2015 KPMG-Plexus.

There is extensive consultation with professional bodies, employers, universities, and health insurers through the Advisory Committee on Medical Manpower Planning to secure support. Data it draws on include care use studies, health insurance statistics, public health data, and social trends.[11] On the back of all this, the health ministry decides how many training places to fund.

But does it work? A detailed study by Malou van Greuningen on the management of the supply of GPs points to some impressive results. In 2000 the advisory committee estimated that the unmet demand for GP care was 5%, but by 2010 this was close to zero. The vacancy rate for GPs remained stable at about 1.7 vacancies per hundred GPs, and there was increasing success in graduates completing specialized GP training being able to find an appropriate place to work. There were also slightly more GPs for the population size by 2010.

Unsurprisingly perhaps, van Greuningen found that the planning system took time to adapt to changing circumstances, and having such a centralized system can make it more difficult to address regional labour market difficulties, even in a reasonably small country. But overall the results—for GPs at least—have been strong.

The planning system faces two big challenges. First, it needs to keep pace with growing differentiation in the size and shape of local populations. For example, the south of Limburg province is ageing more rapidly and has a declining popu-lation, while the major cities have growing numbers of foreign-born citizens and single households.[12] The system also needs to cope with both the high degree of medical specialization and a growing tendency of tasks to shift between profes-sional groups and health organizations in the face of new care practices and cost pressures.[13]

Between 2000 and 2014 there was a 48% increase in medical specialists, far higher than other groups of doctors. But the fastest growing parts of the healthcare work-force were midwives (89%) and occupational therapists, who more than doubled. Hospital nurses increased by more than a third, and there were significant increases in nurses working in care homes and in-home care.[14]

The success of workforce planning for doctors and the requirement for healthcare professionals to speak Dutch means the Netherlands is less dependent on doctors and nurses from other countries than many of its European neighbours; high stand-ards of English mean that the country is a net exporter of staff. However, foreign-trained doctors make a significant contribution to some medical specialties, notably anaesthesiology.

Few nurses come from abroad, even though the number of vacancies increased by about 17% between 2015 and 2017. Some hospitals have suffered such acute shortages that they have been temporarily forced to stop admitting patients.[15] Care homes have also experienced serious shortages. The problem was exacerbated by a tightening of the rules around nursing registration, which removed nurses from the register who had had insufficient training or patient contact in recent years.

Planning for the nursing workforce is considerably less sophisticated than for doc-tors, which may partially explain why there have been more recent difficulties with current nurse vacancies standing at approximately 70,000. But estimates of supply and demand are still used to tweak the number of training places each year. Control of the nursing labour market is devolved to the regions. In line with other industries, there are discussions between employers and unions about the size and shape of the workforce, and there can be some central funding to support initiatives such as training for a specific sector. Pay levels are set nationally, although there is some limited ability to provide local incentives such as a sign-on payment for a GP coming to a sparsely populated area.

Conclusion

The examples of Buurtzorg and an increasing number of other providers in the Netherlands show the power of blurring the distinction between healthcare and social care. Keeping older people and others with high care needs living in their own homes as independently as possible for as long as possible is a model of what good care should be—focused on the needs of the individual and delivered in a way which motivates, develops, and retains the staff.

It might seem somewhat counter-intuitive to pay a bit more for nurses and allied health professionals and then ask them to do everything for patients from the basics to advanced clinical practice, but it works. Across the world, there is a broader ques-tion about the most suitable skill-mix for these type of care needs. Over time, I think the pioneering work of Buurtzorg may well spawn new healthcare providers that allow nurses and allied health professionals to practice at the top of their licence but also introduce care assistants and others into the wider care team as technology advances. I say this because I think the sheer volume of elderly patients and increasing sophistication of digital power will make it both necessary and irresistible.

Finally, the Dutch are also to be applauded for developing a medical workforce planning system which has the confidence of politicians, the professions, employers, universities, and insurers and which delivers clear benefits for patients and taxpayers. Learning from the shortcomings in workforce management which became apparent in the 1990s they wisely decided to construct an approach which could be run and refined over the long term rather than resort to short-term fixes, while the emphasis on well-resourced primary care contributes to outcomes which are impressive by international standards. There is much more to do for nursing and allied health professionals but there is a lot to learn from the Netherlands. It's a very smart country.

Chapter 9

Germany—happy families?

The Germans are proud of their health system and created the first social insurance funds in the world. In 1883 Chancellor Otto von Bismarck established 'sickness funds' which form the foundation of their healthcare today. Back then average life expectancy was under 40 but that has more than doubled, standing at 81 today. Indeed, Germany is projected to have the second highest proportion (23%) by 2021 of citizens aged over 65 and is about to reach a national milestone of having more people aged 60 and over than under 30.[1] This demographic pressure is forcing radical experimentation, with the government paying families to care for their elderly. It will prove to be a test bed for other countries and is worth watching carefully.

Numbers are not enough

Germany spends a lot on healthcare. At 11.2%[2] of gross domestic product (GDP), few other European countries spend as much, and it is not hard to see where it goes. With 4.2 doctors and 12.8 nurses per 1,000 inhabitants,[3] Germany's clinical staffing levels compare very favourably with the European average (Fig. 9.1).

Until recently Germany was in the enviable position of having too many doctors rather than too few. A prevailing belief that access to the career of one's choice should be a right, coupled with a lack of centralized health workforce planning in this federated country, meant that for years the focus of federal government health policy was to curb the resulting supplier-induced demand.[4]

Now it is short of staff because of undersupply, maldistribution and, crucially, because the German health system simply does too much. It sees more, admits more, and treats more than the average Organisation for Economic Co-operation and Development (OECD) country and as its population grows, ages, and expects more it is increasingly struggling to keep up.

In 2015, Germany performed 299 hip replacements per 100,000 population compared with an OECD average of 166,[5] and the hospital discharge rate (measuring the number of patients discharged after a night's care per 100,000 population) is the highest in the OECD.[6] These high activity rates are not all down to clinical need and patient choice.

Successive reforms to try to curb high levels of activity have suffered major setbacks. Although there are pockets of innovation across the country, diffusion is stymied by a fragmented and federated system, and Germany's clinical leaders remain traditional in their approach to care and professional roles.

The German health system has become increasingly reliant on migrant professionals to plug workforce gaps. In 2015, foreign-trained doctors accounted for 11% of those practising—up from 4% in 2000—and 30% of newly registered physicians.[7]

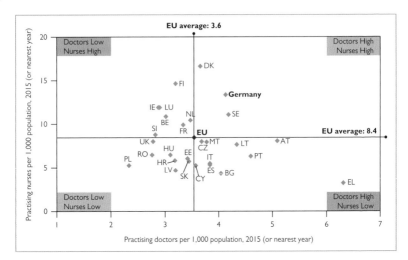

Fig. 9.1 Germany has comparatively high numbers of physicians and nurses for its population.
Reproduced with permission from European Commission. State of Health in the EU—Germany Country Health Profile 2017. Copyright © OECD and World Health Organization.

Rural and less affluent regions lack doctors and there is an acute shortage of nursing staff for older people and those in long-term care.

Migration

German health workers report increasingly high levels of burnout, and every year a growing number of doctors and nurses emigrate, citing workload, pay, and bureaucracy.[8] More doctors leave Germany to work abroad each year than arrive. Accurate figures are difficult to source but we know that about 1% of all active medical doctors left the country in 2008, mostly for German-speaking countries such as Switzerland and Austria.[9] Nurse migration is also on the rise, often to Switzerland and Sweden.

The high number leaving makes the system more reliant on foreign-trained doctors and nurses. Eastern and Central Europe are the most common sources along with Italy and Greece in more recent years. European enlargement in the early 2000s prompted a spike, and the financial crisis of 2008 prompted a second.[10]

However, while more doctors leave Germany than arrive each year, the opposite is true for care workers. Few German citizens move abroad to practise as care workers compared with the numbers arriving. Again, Central and Eastern Europe are key sources.

Germany has had trouble recruiting trained care staff domestically because of poor pay and conditions. According to Destatis, Germany's Federal Office for Statistics, full-time carers receive around €18 an hour compared with the average hourly rate in Germany of €22,[11] a fact that has prompted plans for legislated wage increases from health minister Jens Spahn. Technically, trainees earn as they learn—but only little—and training takes three years. Those attending private schools must pay for their training, although recent legislation promises to abolish the fee from 2020. That may make training places easier to fill but attrition rates are high, with many students quitting the programme as the reality of workloads and staff shortages becomes clear.

German terms and conditions are good, however, compared with Central and Eastern Europe. The average wage in Poland is just over €1,000 a month, whereas in Germany care workers receive upwards of €1,500.[12] In 2005, Germany negotiated bilateral agreements with several Central and Eastern European countries including Poland, Romania, and Croatia for the recruitment of nursing assistants for elderly long-term care.

Germany's reliance on migrant labour has been criticised for depriving source countries of their skills, and now it only negotiates agreements with countries that have excess health workers in accordance with the World Health Organization's Global Code of Practice.[13] For example, it now has an established agreement with the Philippines to recruit nurses, and in 2013 it piloted a bilateral agreement with Vietnam to train nurses to live and work in Germany. One hundred nurses have now come through the scheme and it has been seen as a positive step towards more ethical overseas recruitment.[14]

Long-term care

Despite high rates of care worker immigration, Germany still has persistently high rates of care worker vacancies. It is estimated that for every 100 vacancies there are just 22 job seekers, and in some places that number can be as low as 13.[15]

Mandatory long-term care insurance (LTCI), introduced in 1995, aimed to ease pressure on formal carers by strengthening informal care at home. It was presented as a new deal between citizen and state, with far greater responsibility placed on families to care for their loved ones into older age.[16] In return families could expect some help with the costs of providing that care from the state, though that help was never intended to be comprehensive. Even when state help is provided for residential care costs the only contribution is to the cost of care, not the so-called hotel costs.

As I described in the chapter on patients as partners (Chapter 7), LTCI offered a choice for beneficiaries of either services-in-kind, cash payments, or a mixture of the two. Cash payment was a popular choice, with about two-thirds of beneficiaries choosing that option despite its value being only half that of service-only benefits. This is one way in which the insurance policy was able to be so effective at reducing government care costs. Between 1995 and 1998 the number of people requiring social assistance for long-term care from the state just about halved as home care increased and use of residential care was delayed.[17]

As well as families providing care themselves however, private homecare workers have become an increasingly important source of support for beneficiaries and their families. It seems those with the highest needs are most likely to employ private care workers. Some workers are employed formally, others illegally. Many are migrants. A study by Lutz and Palenga-Mollenbeck (2010) estimated somewhere between 150,000 and 200,000 informal carers were working in Germany at the time[18]: 'women from Central and Eastern Europe shuttling back and forth between their country of origin and the one in which they work'.

Care worker vacancies are still rife, however, and more recently German health minister Jens Spahn announced plans to recruit 8,000 more staff from abroad (particularly Kosovo and Albania), and around 5,000 more from home.[19] But German charities estimate an additional 100,000 are needed to cover current and future care needs. Migrant recruitment cannot possibly fill this gap, not least because of how controversial that would be. To attract more Germans into the job, pay and conditions would have to improve. The plan, 'Konzierte Aktion Pflege' aims to do this, though they may find they need to dig a bit deeper to attract home-grown recruits.

Doing too much

Overactivity has been a worry for successive governments, and for at least the last 40 years there have been repeated reforms of the health system to try to address the issue. There have been restrictions on medical school places and physician posts and reforms to encourage bundled payments, gatekeeping, and accountable care.[20] But although the reforms have produced pockets of exemplar practice, nationwide implementation has proved difficult.

This is partly due to the federated nature of the country. Germany is divided into 16 Länder with many of the key decision-making powers devolved to regional non-governmental bodies. These bodies, which include insurers, doctors' representatives, and hospital federations, negotiate implementation of national policies locally and decide on a wide range of issues from benefits and prices to care standards. All the bodies have vested interests, often conflicting with federal policy, and are in conflict with each other. Legislation to strengthen primary care, for example, has met with much resistance from specialists and hospital providers over the years, muting the impact of most of those policies.

Doctor knows best

Development of new approaches to care is also held back by an antiquated approach to professional roles. It has a highly doctor-centric health system, with German law defining physicians as the leading professional group in the healthcare sector. As such, physicians hold a lot of power. For example, there is little task-shifting to date in Germany and there are only a few opportunities for advanced practice. Doctors are the only clinicians involved in negotiations about services at regional level and they have resisted attempts to delegate tasks and responsibilities to nurses or medical assistants in outpatient care. Non-physicians may only deliver diagnostic or therapeutic services if sanctioned by a physician and only doctors have the power to refer patients to non-physician services. All this has made it hard to develop comprehensive primary care services.

Some national reforms have been successful. The problem of regional imbalances was addressed by a system in which Länder with an oversupply of physicians refused licences to open new treatment centres when saturation reached 110%—effectively establishing a 'one in, one out' policy for outpatient services. Reforms in 2013 also offered family doctors in physician-rich areas full reimbursement for the sale of their business if they were prepared to work in an under-doctored region for five years, and some places offered GPs of retirement age an additional €1,500 per quarter to prolong their tenure in an under-doctored region.

At first glance, the convoluted landscape of regional health workforce planning looks impenetrable to collaborative working, but in Rhineland-Palatinate they are piloting a tool to do just that. The monitoring tool collects workforce data from providers in the region and correlates it with health system outcomes to generate suggestions for changes to education and training programmes. Over time the tool has been learning, and its estimates are getting more accurate. One of the selling points of this tool is that it relies heavily on stakeholder involvement—it is through iterative discussions and evaluations with regional stakeholders that an assessment of the healthcare outcomes is gained and is intrinsic to how the system learns.[21]

Although labour intensive, it has ensured a degree of constructive engagement from stakeholders not previously seen and provided a forum for interprofessional discussions about skill mix, task-shifting, and coordination. This kind of collaborative approach to Germany's regional workforce planning is just what it needs to achieve an evidence-based, needs-based integrated workforce plan.

Conclusion

Germany invests well in its healthcare, runs it smoothly, and secures good outcomes. However, its frenetic activity levels are unnecessary and unsustainable, while its traditional approach to professional roles will exacerbate staff shortages and inhibit the development of badly needed new care models.

But its bold experimentation—at scale—with carers' pay schemes shows great promise, and could demonstrate to other developed countries how to invert the relationship between the state, its elders, and their carers. For a country that often prides itself on its pragmatism it is quietly revolutionary.

Ironically, for a country that sits near the top of the G7 productivity league table, it is odd that traditional role demarcations in healthcare have not evolved. As the most powerful economic force in the European Union, Germany has mastered industrial and manufacturing process re-engineering into a fine art. Its long-term investments in infrastructure and equipment is second to none and its vocational education and highly effective apprenticeships are world-class. Its labour–management relationships are mature and the general commitment to worker well-being and work-life balance are progressive. Sadly, some of these characteristics have somewhat evaded the German healthcare industry to date but it is only a matter of time before the potential is realized.

Chapter 10

The professions—on top of their game?

When I joined the UK's National Health Service (NHS) Management Training Scheme 30 years ago, a distinguished doctor sat me down and told me that the wonderful thing about healthcare was that all of humanity could be found within it: 'From porters to professors, patients to politicians and the public to the press, the best and worst in life and death can be found in healthcare.' He wasn't wrong—health professionals are some of the most caring, dedicated, and talented people I have ever met. In a world increasingly obsessed by celebrity and fame, they represent all that is decent in humankind. No wonder a recent global Organisation for Economic Co-operation and Development (OECD) survey of students found that a career in the health profession was ranked first. People join healthcare through a strong vocation, but we often take this for granted when it should be continually nurtured.

Poor systems and bad organization make a tough job stressful and unproductive. They sap the joy from what health professionals are doing and shamefully undervalue the time, money, and effort that they (and the system) have invested—especially when they quit.

We funnel people into specialisms and then deprive them of the support they need to do their job. We make it hard for people to transfer from one specialism to another. We train people in skills that will become obsolete and fail to give them skills they will need their entire career. We fail to match skills to patients' changing needs. In addition, we control all this through workforce policies which hope for certainty instead of planning for adaptability.

This is not fair on anybody. We can manage and lead the clinical professions better than this. In some places, they do. This chapter is about how we realize that potential—through education, training, teamwork, and technology—and harness the best we can from people as individuals and in teams.

Productive people

Individual clinicians are capable of more and they know it. The OECD has assembled compelling evidence from doctors and nurses in many countries of the level of 'skills mismatch' between what they have and what they need, while 76% of doctors and 79% of nurses have reported performing tasks for which they were overqualified (Fig. 10.1).[1,2]

Tasks nurses find themselves doing include delivering food, transporting patients around the hospital, cleaning patients' rooms and equipment, and collecting supplies. Administrative tasks are another bugbear. In the United Kingdom, the Royal College

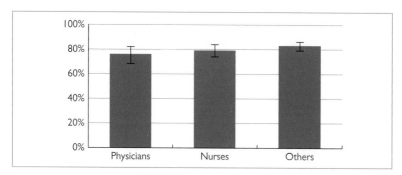

Fig. 10.1 Reported overskilling by physicians, nurses, and other occupations, PIAAC survey, 2011/2012. Reproduced with permission from Buchan, J. et al. (Eds). Health Employment and Economic Growth: An Evidence Base. Geneva, Switzerland: World Health Organization. Copyright © 2017 WHO.

of Nursing estimates that around 18% of nursing time is spent on 'non-essential' paperwork,[3] and the British Medical Association reports trainee doctors spend around 15% of their time doing the same thing. In the United States it is thought to be one of the driving forces behind physician burnout.

So the first challenge is helping professionals to work at the limits of their licence— and ensuring that every member of the healthcare team knows what those limits are is a good place to start. PACK (the Practical Approach to Care Kit) is a handbook of evidence-based treatment pathways for the management of common conditions in primary care. It was devised by a South African respiratory physician in the 1990s in response to the high number of patients he was seeing with complications of respiratory diseases that might have been prevented or managed better in the community. Apart from setting out much clearer diagnostic, management, and referral guidelines for the primary health team, PACK also colour-coded every step to help each professional in the team identify which of them had the authority to carry out each task. Subsequent evaluations showed that this gave those professionals more confidence to work at the limits of their licence, boosting productivity and effectiveness. PACK was so successful it was eventually absorbed into the South African primary healthcare programme and has since been expanded to other countries in Africa and South America.[4]

Redesigning care pathways is another way to make better use of professionals' time. In India a group of cancer treatment centres called HealthCare Global (HCG) configure their facilities in a 'hub and spoke' network. Their most highly trained oncologists, pathologists, and surgeons work out of three hubs in Ahmedabad, Mumbai, and Chennai, and their super-specialists out of a super-hub in Bangalore. Specialists carry out the most complex procedures using equipment such as cyclotrons, linear accelerators and, in the super-hub, a Cyberknife robotic radiosurgery system. Image sharing and telemedicine technology allows these specialists to remain in the hub where their services are more productively employed, but continue to provide expert advice to the 18 spoke facilities where most diagnosis, treatment, and follow-up care is provided.[5]

Operational excellence like this can be a powerful tool for unlocking productivity but is often controversial with staff. World leaders in these techniques like Virginia Mason Medical Center in Seattle are well aware of the need for strong clinical input, leadership, and buy-in to make changes like this effective and sustainable.

Virginia Mason is known for its application of the Toyota production system, but its work in changing the relationship between the organization and its doctors—the human side of the system—is just as impressive. For example, it organized a retreat for physicians and managers which gave physicians the opportunity to talk candidly about their frustrations and the whole group the chance to debate what a new compact between the organization and its staff should look like. This triggered months of work encompassing both enthusiasts and sceptics. Department meetings were held in which the draft compact was discussed, revised, and eventually approved. The final document established reciprocal expectations between Virginia Mason and its physicians. A few chose to leave, but the widespread support for the compact meant that both parties shared a vision of Virginia Mason as a quality leader in healthcare. This unity of purpose enabled the medical centre's ambitious improvement programmes to succeed, building on the willingness of their clinicians to exploit their skills to the full.

At the Aravind Eye Hospital in Madurai, which I described in the chapter on India (Chapter 3), ophthalmic surgeons only ever perform that part of the operation that requires their presence. Everything else—from screening and transporting patients to hospital to preparing them for surgery and even follow-up care—is provided by support staff. As a result, while US ophthalmic surgeons average around 400 surgeries a year, Aravind surgeons perform more than 1,000.

The knock-on effect on cost is staggering. Aravind operates at just 1% of the cost of the NHS, and that is by no means simply down to lower pay. For Aravind, productivity gains like these have meant it can treat most of its patients for free or at heavily subsidized rates. And this is high-quality care—complication rates at Aravind are about half that of the United Kingdom.[6]

Meanwhile, in Colorado, a primary care initiative called APEX (Ambulatory Process Excellence) employs medical assistants to support clinicians. They take a history from the patient, present to the physician or nurse, document the appointment, and stay on to provide the patient with health coaching and education. Within six months burnout rates among clinicians dropped from 53% to 13%, and despite the increased cost of hiring additional staff, productivity gains made the intervention cost neutral, with doctors seeing an average of three more patients each day.[7]

Support does not have to come in human form. Microsoft has designed a technology it hopes will take over at least one administrative task—note taking. Scribe is artificial intelligence (AI)-enabled software that can listen to, interpret, write, and code the doctor–patient consultation, reducing the administrative burden, and cutting consultation times. The potential of exponential technologies like these (that is, innovations that stimulate productivity rather than add to demand) will end up reshaping the clinical workforce.

Advanced practice

Beyond the limits of existing scopes of practice, professionals across the globe have shown how much more they are capable of when properly trained and supported. Extended roles can mean anything from taking on one new responsibility—such as nurse prescribing—to stepping into a new professional space, such as where there are staff shortages in rural areas.

Nurses in Mozambique have been trained to provide emergency obstetric care while community health workers in South Africa diagnose and manage HIV. Many countries are now re-examining the traditional functions of health professionals. Between 2007 and 2012 about half of the OECD countries expanded the scope of practice for non-physician providers such as nurse practitioners and pharmacists,[8] and in Canada, the Netherlands, and the United States education programmes for advanced nurse practitioners are expanding.

In the wake of the European Working Time Directive and mandatory capping of junior doctors' hours, Sheffield Teaching Hospitals NHS Foundation Trust in the United Kingdom was finding it hard to fill junior doctor rota gaps. So it developed a programme to train other professionals in the hospital to fill those roles as advanced clinical practitioners (ACPs).[9] The programme was successful and last year, North Cumbria University Hospitals NHS Trust went further, training five ACPs to become Senior ACPs in acute care medicine.[10] Their two-year training programme follows the Royal College of Physicians' curriculum and will see graduates emerge as middle grades working alongside conventionally trained medical registrars in the hospital in a part of the country that had struggled to recruit.

Primary care nurse practitioners are an example of a partial substitution role. Again, necessity being the mother of invention, it was a shortage of physicians in rural areas of the United States that prompted the introduction of this role. There is now 50 years of evidence to support the safety and effectiveness of nurse practitioners, particularly in the diagnosis and treatment of acute minor ailments and chronic long-term conditions. The level of substitution depends on the degree to which nurses are regulated in each state, with the highest level of substitution by those nurses who are able both to work autonomously and prescribe. A paper by Dubois and Singh in 2009 estimates that advanced practice nurses can handle about 70% of a GP's work-load.[11] In the Netherlands, workforce models project that a reallocation of tasks from GPs to nurse practitioners will reduce demand for GPs by 0.6–1.2% per year, while modelling in Switzerland forecasts that task substitution could slow the growth in GP consultations from 13% to 2%.[12] So the gains are significant.

In the United Kingdom, extended scope physiotherapists are taking on greater roles in musculoskeletal services. Where patients are able to self-refer, the service can relieve the workload of GPs. Where physiotherapists are able to triage and treat, they can reduce the burden on specialists.

At some point this task-shifting between professionals inevitably meets resistance. We came up against physician resistance in the United Kingdom in 2006 when we introduced nurse prescribing and over a decade later, we are meeting it again from registered nurses, some of whom object to the introduction of nursing associates. Even the term task-shifting brings out antibodies in people who think it is workforce expansion on the cheap or delegating the jobs you don't like (pejoratively referred to as 'task-shafting').

Workforce policy analyst Dr Patricia Oakley understands the process can be uncomfortable: 'Clever strategic workforce planning understands the inter- and intraprofessional tensions and rivalry and uses new technology and AI to shift the boundaries and thus the areas of control and their worth. You can take the Abbott line[13]—it's a system and you have to work it to change things—or the Krause line[14] where it's about trade and monopolies. Either way, this is the intellectual underpinning to strategic workforce planning if you want to create a more flexible workforce.'

Task-shifting is not always successful. The Ministry of Health in Mozambique suspended training of non-physician clinicians employed to provide antiretroviral therapy (ART) to HIV patients due to the poor quality of care results—although similar projects elsewhere have had good results. It is important to understand whether a project has failed as a proof of concept or because of problems with implementation—the right training, support, and so on—and for that, you need data.

Even then, data needs to be interpreted carefully. For example, the recent RN4CAST study of nursing across Europe found that substituting one nursing assistant for a registered nurse on a ward was associated with a 21% increase in the odds of a patient dying[15]—which is shocking, but that is not what I am advocating. Task-shifting is about ratios of staff as well as absolute numbers, and in healthcare it is more often about supplementing and complementing than replacing. It is entirely possible that both more nurses and more nursing assistants are required simultaneously.

Task-shifting is sometimes unfairly dismissed as cost-*in*effective. True, the evidence for cost-effectiveness of nurse-led clinics, for example, is equivocal; appointment times are often that bit longer and referral rates slightly higher. However, their clinical outcomes are the same and to look at the cost-effectiveness of one service in isolation is to miss the point. The real value is in the difference it makes to the productivity of the system, not the service.

Finally, task-shifting may not always be appropriate. For example, there are cases where task-shifting has led to fragmentation of care. District nursing in the Netherlands 10 years ago is a case in point. In an effort to cut costs, nursing duties were contracted out to separate providers, each trained only to the minimum level required to carry out that task. Different carers would come to wash the patient, serve meals, or put on elastic compression stockings and the overall quality of care was poor. That's what prompted Jos de Blok to launch Buurtzorg in 2007 with district nurses able to do everything for the patient from washing and dressing to putting up intravenous lines at home.[16] The service cost more per hour to provide but patients found they needed far fewer hours, about a third less, in part because nurses had been given the autonomy to solve the patient's problems holistically rather than just executing fixed tasks and leaving. Context is important.

'Top of your game' versus 'top of your capacity'

There is a distinction to be made between working at the top of your game and just being incredibly busy. I am not advocating the latter. Working at full tilt for 12 hours a day with not even enough time to look after yourself, let alone your patients, is a path to burnout. What I am advocating—working at the top of your game—is different. It is doing what only you can do. It means seniors not acting down to cover junior shifts because of rota gaps, letting support staff take on the administrative burden so that clinicians can get on and treat patients, and taking advantage of technology to allow junior staff to take on more responsibility.

Technology driving new roles

Developments in AI, remote monitoring and the Internet of Things will drive this trend towards task-shifting and accelerate the disruption of the current healthcare workforce. We are already starting to see models like this in low- and middle-income countries.

In sub-Saharan Africa, for example, where in rural areas in particular there are few clinicians for the population size, community health workers are increasingly assisted by portable technology to bridge the gap. The area of medical need where mobile technology seems to have taken off is antenatal and postnatal health for mothers and babies—and that need is great. Across the globe almost 300,000 women a year die from obstetric causes and 3.3 million children are stillborn. A further 3.3 million die within the first month of life.[17] Most of those deaths would be preventable with cost-effective interventions but 99% of them occur in countries where access to help is limited.

The community health workers in people's homes and remote clinics are using smartphone technology such as up-to-date evidence and advice for expectant parents, protocols for assessing and triaging patients, clinical decision support tools, access to remote specialist advice, the ability to upload still and video images for review, the potential to connect additional sensors and devices, global positioning services, and drug calculation tools. To date, I'm not aware of a system that does the lot, but it can't be long.

Simple interventions can be highly effective. A study of pregnant women in Zanzibar found that access to a text and phone advice service called Wired Mums halved perinatal mortality.[18] However, not all interventions are tested or validated, and tech companies have been criticised for targeting poorer countries to pilot their apps because of a dearth of regulation and oversight. Governments have a crucial role in regulating this market and integrating it with existing health systems.

Nonetheless, the implications of this kind of technology are clear. The capacity of health workers with much less formal training to support the scarce resource of doctors and nurses is vast. I predict this cadre of workers will grow the fastest in the next decade, although we will need to tread carefully into this uncharted territory.

Planning for technological change

Yet despite the profound changes which technology is driving, I have yet to see anyone in health get a grip on the impact of automation on workforce planning. Organizations and systems seem to be letting technology happen to them rather than thinking creatively about how to prepare for it. Figure 10.2 illustrates just some of the questions healthcare leaders need to be asking.

Other industries have been far quicker off the mark. The insurance industry is a case in point. KPMG has recently completed a piece of work for a major insurer helping them to assess the extent to which automation might affect the size and shape of their workforce in future and what they can do to prepare for this. By prepare, I don't mean lay off workers—I mean figure out where their experienced and highly skilled workers might be better deployed in future and what training they might need to get there.

To complete this piece of work, we collaborated with Imperial College Data Observatory who have developed a tool called Foo.castr—a piece of software that takes job descriptions, breaks roles down into tasks, and then identifies what proportion of those tasks might be automated in future. This enables organizations to see which departments and which professions might be most affected and helps plan their business accordingly. The results are unique to a business—not just the industry.

No one has ever tried this with healthcare until now but last year, Imperial College Data Observatory started work with University Hospitals Birmingham NHS

Key questions that will shape the workforce

— What is the art of the possible with digital technology?
— What skills and capabilities are needed in your organization in the next two to five years?
— Which organization models and structures achieve the best integration of human and intelligent automation?
— How should organizations integrate contingent workers with permanent core employees?
— What is the moral and ethical framework that leaders wish to work within in relation to workforce displacement, transition and replacement?
— How can the existing (human) workforce expand the scope of its current role in the organization to provide value-added services beyond the scope of the bots?
— How can organizations develop a comprehensive strategy to reform the education and training system to be more responsive to demands of the future workforce?
— How can organizations redesign their current job profiles to attract, retain, and absorb future talent with advanced technological skills?
— Out of the many emerging technologies claiming to automate work, which ones will work in the context of your organization—and which ones are not applicable, or simply hype?

Fig. 10.2 Key questions that will shape the workforce.

Foundation Trust to analyse the impact automation could have on the clinical and administrative workforce of their cancer and COPD services and the implications that had for service delivery.

We are now almost a decade into the fourth industrial revolution and productivity, rather than skyrocketing, has slowed to an almost crawling pace.

The productivity lag was, to a certain extent, expected. Each of the three industrial revolutions before it saw the same and it even has a name—the productivity paradox. The issue, it is thought, is that incumbent managers fail to recognize the potential of technology as it emerges and may adopt it, but replicate the same tired production processes. Five to ten years later, a new cohort of managers arrives and asks 'Why have we always done it like this?'

Josh Bersin of Deloitte gives the example of production line automation. Initially, machines replaced people but when they broke down and production lines snarled up, it didn't save much time at all. Henry Ford saw the potential in these new machines and his five insights into production line processing (subdivision of labour, interchangeable parts, single function machines, sequential ordering of machines, and automatic movement of the produced good) revolutionized the assembly line. Between 1910 and 1920 the price of Ford cars fell by 75%, the number of cars produced rose 5,000%, and Ford employees got a 100% pay rise.[19]

Professional development

The trend towards roles with less formal training in no way detracts from the need to invest in further education and training of the health workforce. Access to continuing professional development (CPD) is a vital prerequisite to the advanced practice of health professionals. CPD is the focus of postgraduate, in-service training that allows professionals to keep their skills up to date and in line with local health needs.

Sometimes countries are misled into thinking that providing the training is enough. To be truly effective, parallel changes in regulation, legislation, and employment are required to ensure newly learned skills are translated into safe, effective practice. There is no point, for example, putting on a nurse-prescribing course if nurse prescribing is not legal. Similarly, when changes to education and legislation occur, failure to adjust regulation can mute their impact. In the United Kingdom, for example, physician assistants remain unregulated, leaving many practices reticent about taking them on to work autonomously.

It is important that health professionals can see the employment opportunities at the other end of that training. Kenya has been criticised for expanding access to medical education without simultaneously expanding the number of posts on graduation, leading to underemployment of doctors in a system which has high unmet need. Similarly, efforts internationally to guide medical graduates into primary care have been undermined by a failure to make the positions more attractive.

Attractiveness does not have to mean higher wages. When Ireland introduced nurse prescribing in 2006 there was no pecuniary benefit to nurses in completing the course but that did not stop it being wildly successful. According to Ireland's chief nursing officer it was the ability to get on and provide the service they wanted to give that drove them.

Pluri-potential staff

CPD can also be a means to greater flexibility in the workforce. When clinicians gain accreditation for new knowledge and skills, those competencies become transferrable. This is called credentialing and is potentially valuable over time as roles change. In the United Kingdom the General Medical Council has piloted its use for breast disease management and musculoskeletal medicine,[20] the idea being to provide the public with assurance of doctors' standards in new and emerging areas of medical practice while avoiding the 'snakes and ladders' of rigid training schemes and fossilized job descriptions.

Credentialing may also be of value when responsibilities are lost from roles. For example, radiology looks set to lose significant chunks of what today would be bread and butter tasks of the job. If suddenly fewer radiologists were required, credentialing might allow them to take their transferrable skills into a different area of medicine such as surgery or emergency medicine, without having to spend seven more years retraining and covering old ground. Just because a role becomes redundant, it does not mean the clinician has to follow it.

Given how difficult it is to predict what the needs of health systems in years to come might be, CPD and credentialing in particular offer the opportunity for clinicians to be permanently pluripotential staff—like stem cells they could be anything they want (or you need them) to be.

Productive teams

Task-shifting will have a profound impact on the ratio of health professionals required to optimize productivity. The Health Foundation found a striking correlation between consultant productivity and nurse to consultant ratios in teams up and down the United Kingdom. On average, each 4% increase in nursing numbers compared with consultants was associated with a 1% increase in consultant productivity.[21]

Getting these ratios right presents something of a difficulty for workforce planners. Not only do they face decisions now about the numbers of professionals needed 10 or 15 years hence, but those numbers and ratios are almost certainly going to change over time as technology and medicine evolve. Workforce planning means aiming at a moving target.

The kind of forecasting required to look 10–15 years into the future would take a crystal ball but it does not mean that health systems can't plan at all—they just need to be both tactical and strategic. Some things are more certain than others. We know exactly, for example, what is happening to the burden of disease across the globe—the same tide of chronic illness and multimorbidity has now crashed against the shores of almost every country as they ride the wave of the epidemiological shift. Similarly, health systems globally are moving towards a primary care led, integrated model.

On the other hand, technology is a much lesser known quantity and demand for skills can change quickly. A number of years ago, the United Kingdom invested heavily in training cardiothoracic surgeons to carry out coronary artery bypass graft procedures for heart attacks. Almost immediately, the advent of angioplasty and stenting made those skills redundant.

Workforce planning is not an exact science. It can set a broad direction but there needs to be give in the system, and that means iterative planning and an agile workforce that can respond to changes in the medical and technical landscape.

It also needs to be coordinated across the professions. A recent report by the Health Foundation laid bare what can happen to workforce productivity when different professions grow asymmetrically. Between 2010 and 2016, the UK consultant workforce grew by over 20% while nursing numbers grew by just 1.6%, resulting in a 2.3% year on year decline in consultant productivity.[22]

Across the globe, there seems to be a broad consensus between planners that the skill mix of the future will be much more weighted towards the ranks of staff such as nurses, nursing assistants, and care workers rather than medical specialists. For example, workforce modelling by the England's Department of Health and Social Care predicts a much higher ratio of nurses to doctors in the next 20–25 years, and an even higher ratio of allied staff to nurses. This certainly mirrors what I have seen in high-performing organizations. At Aravind Eye Hospital, for example, there are six auxiliary clinical staff and four administrative assistants for every surgeon, and in Colorado, when they introduced the medical assistants for primary care physicians as part of its APEX scheme, the ratio of medical assistants to clinicians grew from 1:1 to 2.5:1.[23] Brazil and its Programa Saude da Familia (Family Health Programme) is another obvious example of this in primary care.

But while planning for different staff ratios is one thing, and probably best done from a top-down perspective, dealing with the nitty gritty of task reallocation between team members is another, and almost certainly needs to come from the bottom upwards. This is where Human Resources Information Systems (HRIS) could come into their own. Future HRIS are looking to triangulate data on staff ratios, patient outcomes, and productivity to provide a more evidence-based approach to workforce planning and, eventually, learning health systems. HRIS are considered so valuable that the World Health Organization has developed its own—iHRIS—that is freely available for countries to download and use. However, despite claiming to be the only class of hospital information system that benefits both care and costs,[24] HRIS are still something of a Cinderella, perpetually in the shadow of their more glamorous sister the clinical information system, and often failing to get the interest and investment they deserve.[25]

Ambition

There is immense untapped talent in our workforce and a lot of inefficiency. In 2010 the World Health Report estimated that between 20 and 40% of global health spending was wasted, with the health workforce representing a substantial portion of that.[26] Organizational ambition, creative thinking, technological innovation, a focus on matching skills to tasks and emphasizing lifelong professional development over preservice training have huge potential to get every professional to the top of their game and, by doing so, allow others into healthcare. Let's work smarter, not harder.

Chapter 11

Loving your staff—bring joy to work

When the United States joined the Second World War in 1941, demand for steel soared. One steel production plant, in Oakland California, swelled to 90,000 employees as they struggled to generate enough steel for local shipbuilding operations. Steel production was not as health and safety conscious then as it is now and the company often lost workers' time through sickness and injury. To keep them healthy and productive, the steel company set up a hospital and health facilities nearby and provided the service as a benefit to its employees. After the war ended, demand for steel declined and the production plant eventually went out of business but the health facilities remained. The steel company was called Kaiser Industries. The health business is what we now know as Kaiser Permanente.

Good employers have long understood the benefits to productivity of happy, healthy staff, and retaining, engaging, and motivating staff are key to any workforce strategy. Clinicians are expensive to train and it takes years. Once lost, they are not easily replaced. Yet we lose people from their first day in the job.

They might quit because of the job itself or through personal circumstances. But if health systems want to retain people throughout their working lives, they are going to have to support them through life events—births, deaths, parenthood, sickness, caring, older age. And they will have to support them through every stage of their career too, from first job, through promotion and into retirement. They are also, like any other industry, going to have to meet legitimate expectations of a healthy, happy relationship with work.

Without it, people disengage, cut back hours, migrate, take early retirement, and take more time off sick. Not only is this bad news for countries with a workforce crisis, it is also bad news for individual employers. The cost to the employer of nurse turnover is estimated to be up to double the salary of the person leaving,[1] while a 1% reduction in National Health Service (NHS) absenteeism would save a typical UK hospital trust £1m in frontline agency staff. Companies spend time and effort understanding exactly what their customers want and need of them—it is time healthcare providers started asking that about their workforce.

Unloved

Doctors and nurses globally are feeling a bit unloved, as Figure 11.1 illustrates. A 2016 survey by Merritt Hawkins of 17,000 American doctors for the Physicians Foundation found that 54% reported low morale, 49% would not recommend medicine as a career to their children, and 48% plan to cut back on patient facing hours

Doctors

Rank	Factors	18–25 years	26–35 years	36–45 years	46+ years
1	Work-life balance	Work-life balance	Work-life balance	Work-life balance	Amount of time to engage with patients / Support from immediate team
2	Amount of time to engage with patients	Felxibility of shifts	Recognition / Amount of time to engage with patients	Amount of time to engage with patients	Pay
3	Pay	Pay	Pay	Support from immediate team	Felxibility of shifts / Work-life balance
4	Flexibility of shifts	Opportunities for CPD	Felxibility of shifts / Opportunities for CPD / Support from immediate team	Felxibility of shifts / The support I get from my organization	Level of responsibility
5	Support from immediate team	The support I get from my organization	Level of responsibility / The support I get from my organization	Pay	Recognition / Sense of fulfilment / Opportunities for CPD / The support I get from my organization

Nurses

Rank	Factors	18–25 years	26–35 years	36–45 years	46+ years
1	Pay	Work-life balance	Work-life balance	Pay	Pay
2	Work-life balance	Pay	Pay	Work-life balance	Amount of time to engage with patients / Work-life balance
3	Felxibility of shifts	Felxibility of shifts	Felxibility of shifts	Recognition / Support from immediate team	Felxibility of shifts
4	Amount of time to engage with patients	Amount of time to engage with patients	Amount of time to engage with patients	Amount of time to engage with patients / Flexibility of shifts	Recognition / Support from immediate team
5	Recognition	Recognition	Support from immediate team	Opportunities for CPD	Level of responsibility

Fig. 11.1 Top five drivers of doctors' dissatisfaction and top five drivers of nurses' dissatisfaction. Reproduced with permission from Deloitte. Time to care: securing a future for the hospital workforce in the UK. London, UK: Deloitte Centre for Healthcare Solutions. Copyright © 2018 Deloitte.

or retire. In China, Lo et al. (2018) report incredible physician burnout rates of 66–87%,[2] while in the last two years we have seen doctors striking in India and the United Kingdom.

Nurses aren't faring any better. In 2016 the national survey of nurses and midwives in Australia found that almost a third had considered leaving the profession because of burnout,[3] while a 2012 European study by Aiken et al. found burnout rates in Greek nurses of 78%.[4] Burnout—a syndrome characterized by emotional exhaustion, cynicism, and a low sense of accomplishment—is associated with higher absenteeism and mental illness and worse patient mortality.

Why are healthcare staff the world over feeling so unloved? Factors vary widely. In India and China, for example, violence against doctors has become commonplace, with some Chinese hospitals now employing armed guards to protect physicians.

But despite local differences there are some common themes—workload, pay, flexibility, respect, and career progression all feature highly.

Workload

Probably the most consistent feature is workload. Time to Care, a Deloitte study of doctors and nurses in European hospitals, reported that doctors in 8 out of the 11 countries found their workload more difficult to manage than five years ago. Nurses in 10 of the countries held the same view.[5] Both 'work-life balance' and 'time to engage with patients' topped the scoreboard for job dissatisfaction. The UK's Nursing and Midwifery Council reports that the most common reason given for nurses quitting before retirement is poor working conditions.[6]

In China, doctors also report high workloads. Wu et al.'s 2014 study of doctors in Zhejiang found that provincial hospital doctors had the longest hours, with almost half seeing over 100 patients a day and 60% working 60-hour weeks.[7] As a result many of them had average consultation times of just four minutes—which is actually only just below the global average. According to a 2017 study by Irving et al., half the world's population has a primary care consultation time of less than five minutes. According to the study, the shortest is in Bangladesh—just 48 seconds.[8]

In the United States the biggest source of physician dissatisfaction is administration and regulation. According to the Merritt Hawkins survey, 80% said they were overextended or at capacity and 58% gave regulatory or paperwork burdens as the reason. The report estimates that a fifth of physicians' time is now taken up with non-clinical paperwork and 5% is spent tracking quality indicators for new value-based payment models, such as the one mandated by the 2015 Medicare access legislation known as MACRA.[9]

The intensity chain

Research into workforce shortages in paediatric (and particularly neonatal) doctors in the United Kingdom looks at how doctors have responded to growing workloads resulting from staff shortages. At first staff try to make up the difference, but after a while the intensity of the job gets too much. Some choose to leave but more commonly doctors reduce their hours to self-regulate their work-life balance. This may go largely unnoticed at first (as reduced hours are not recorded as vacancies), but the problem has now reached critical mass in the United Kingdom. Consultant paediatricians end up acting down to cover the shifts of absent junior colleagues and overburdened juniors refer more patients up the intensity chain to reduce their own workload, perpetuating a vicious cycle that can be hard to break.

Pay

Pay is in the top five causes of job dissatisfaction for doctors and nurses in every country in Deloitte's European study, and was the number one complaint in Finland,

Sweden, and Switzerland. Unsurprisingly, it seems to be a bigger issue for nurses than doctors; it was the biggest driver of job dissatisfaction for nurses in the United Kingdom but only the third for doctors. Within Europe and globally it is the most powerful driver of nurse migration.

In China, low levels of physician reimbursement have been blamed for high levels of dual practice—doing two jobs—and supplier-induced demand. A 2016 report by the World Bank, World Health Organization, and Chinese government acknowledged that many primary care doctors in villages had resorted to supplementing their income by selling prescription drugs at high mark-ups, while there has been a problem with hospital doctors charging for unnecessary investigations and treatments, a practice that has fuelled healthcare inflation in China and possibly the rise in attacks on staff.

Careers

Lack of career progression is a source of great discontent for doctors and nurses alike, but particularly for nurses. Advanced nurse practitioners are now a common feature in the United States and parts of Europe, while many countries including Thailand, Uganda, South Africa, and Columbia permit nurse prescribing, but it is still not the case everywhere.

In India, for example, a nurse may work for 25 years in intensive care and still not be allowed to prescribe simple analgesia or give an injection without a doctor present. This is thought to be an important cause of high nurse turnover rates there. Lakshman (2016) reports that the turnover of Indian nurses is 28–35%.[10] Devi Shetty, cardiac surgeon and founder of Narayana Health in India, reports that turnover in some Delhi hospitals is closer to 75%.

In China, research by Yang et al. (2017) report that young nurses are the most dissatisfied, often citing the 'physician-led, nurse assisted' model of care where there is little room for independent clinical activities or career advancement. Nurses still perform many non-nursing tasks.[11]

Career progression can be an issue for doctors too. In 2017, government doctors in the Indian state of Tamil Nadu went on hunger strike to protest against the slashing of postgraduate seat quotas for doctors in government hospitals.[12] In a country where government posts are poorly paid and few, postgraduate seats offer an opportunity to specialize and seek employment in the private sector. Doctors who fail to secure a postgraduate training place often face unemployment and migration is common, especially to Saudi Arabia and other Middle East countries.

Inflexible working

Poor flexibility is a big problem—again, particularly for nurses. In China, part-time working arrangements are rare. Most nursing posts in government hospitals are 40-hour weeks and even changing the hospital you work for is fraught with bureaucracy. Lack of flexibility is the most commonly cited reason UK nurses give for having left the profession when they return after having children and is a common reason to switch to agency work, a practice which comes at a high price for hospitals.

It is not just nurses of childbearing age however; inflexible working rules affect staff who find themselves caring for a relative or who want to wind down closer to retirement. It affects people recovering from illness or who want to take time out to pursue a parallel interest in research, teaching, or management. It also affects millennials. According to Deloitte, inflexible shifts were the biggest cause of job dis-satisfaction after work-life balance for UK doctors aged 18–25.

The distinction between generational outlooks was also marked in the United States. Merritt Hawkins observed a difference between what they called the 'old guard' of physicians (over 46 years old, male, private practice owners, and specialists) and what they describe as the 'new guard' (younger, female, salaried, primary care based). The old guard reported much lower morale and attributed it predominantly to high levels of paperwork, regulatory compliance, and an erosion of clinical autonomy. The new guard were more optimistic, perhaps because the income and influence of primary care physicians has increased under new value-based delivery models and salaried em-ployees are less exposed to new practice management responsibilities.

The US example highlights another, somewhat paradoxical issue, which is the painful transition many health economies are making greater accountability in the care system. In 2017 in the Indian state of Karnataka, 50,000 private doctors went on strike to protest at a bill proposing fixed pricing for procedures in private hospitals, compliance with infrastructure and staffing standards, and new avenues for redress of patients' grievances, including the ability to charge doctors with medical negligence.

To quote Tolstoy, happy families are all alike; every unhappy family is unhappy in its own way. While many of the issues here—pay, regulation, demand—fall outside the remit of what some individual employers can deliver there is still a lot they can do, as demonstrated by big differences between hospitals in the same country in staff satisfaction, turnover, and absenteeism. To love their staff, health employers need to do more than just deal with what is bothering them. They also need to tap into what drives the opposite—job satisfaction.

Health Education England, which oversees workforce policy, says the biggest single cause of the current NHS workforce crisis is deterioration in staff retention. In 2016–2017 it lost 5,000 more nurses for reasons other than retirement than in 2011–2012. If retention had stayed the same since that year, there would be an add-itional 16,000 nurses now working in the NHS—in other words, the current nurse vacancy rate would be halved.[13]

Improving retention means looking at every facet of the work experience, including organizational values and culture, support during the first few weeks and months of starting a job, career planning and development, and flexible working and retire-ment. All this needs to be underpinned by collecting and analysing the right data to identify trends and retention problem hotspots.

Getting the culture right

Culture is tricky to define but it is a strong driver of retention and it does not happen by accident. NextGen, a 2013 PwC report looking at trends in their own millennial workforce, identified a strong link between retention and the emotional connection their employees had with the organization. That connection was determined by their experience of working there, encompassing everything from people and pay through to opportunities and workload—in other words the employee value proposition (EVP).[14] Getting retention right requires a coordinated strategy across all these fronts.

The Magnet Recognition Program in the United States is just such a strategy for nursing. Run by the American Nurses' Credentialing Center (ANCC), an affiliate of the American Nurses Association (ANA), the programme grants Magnet status to hospitals meeting standards of excellence in nursing. The programme was developed in the 1980s after an ANA study of 41 high nurse-retaining hospitals in the United States identified common characteristics. Around 600 hospitals in the United States have Magnet status as well as a handful outside it.

Magnet hospitals have above-average patient outcomes—4.6% lower mortality, for example—while the turnover of non-Magnet hospitals attributable to staffing and workload problems is almost 4.7 times higher.[15]

An independent evaluation by the University of Pennsylvania in 2013 found the programme's success was down to three features: improved nurse to patient staffing ratios; higher nurse education standards; and a better working environment.[16]

Work environment—the organizational characteristics of work—was found to be the most significant factor, and other evidence supports this. Research in the International Journal of Nursing Studies (Hayes et al., 2006) found interventions aimed at improving the environment had a bigger impact on staff retention than increasing recruitment or salaries.[17]

The working environment is not just resources and the physical environment (though they are important). Other features of high nurse-retaining hospitals are: friendly staff, effective management, a higher degree of professional autonomy for nurses, a greater degree of control over their practice setting, a feeling of being listened to and represented by effective nurse leaders, having positive physician–nurse relationships, working in a hospital that promotes the status of nursing, and working for an organization that promotes excellence in patient care and supports nurses through education and training to achieve that.[18]

It is about being professionally and personally valued by patients and colleagues. Putting that into practice is the next step. In 2017 the Institute of Health Improvement launched Joy at Work, an initiative to help health providers tackle burnout and promote engagement by improving the work environment.[19] It is not prescriptive about how to achieve it. Instead, it recommends employers simply ask their employees 'What matters to you?' and then experiment with what works in that organization, using improvement science to track and evaluate impact. It warns against reinventing the wheel, however. There are plenty of evidence-based interventions to run with, such as promoting nurses to hospital executive positions or initiating nurse–physician co-design of clinical protocols.

Frimley Health NHS Foundation Trust in southern England, rated outstanding by inspectors, has demonstrated how putting a big effort into getting the culture right can deliver extraordinary results.[20] In 2014 it took over the nearby Heatherwood and Wexham Park hospitals, which had been struggling. To build a unified culture across the entire group, human resources (HR) and other teams collected data through interviews and questionnaires and compared these with other measures such as staff sickness, recruitment feedback, and staff survey data. This informed a new organizational development strategy and a huge training programme in organizational values. Senior staff were seen to be committed to changing the climate in the newly acquired hospitals and to engage with staff over the long term. The values and behaviours which had become embedded successfully at Frimley Park were tested at the new hospitals to see how they would be accepted, and some adjustments were made.

Around 600 line managers received training on customer care and values, and 700 on leadership. To improve culture further, members of the senior management team are based across all sites and role model the values and behaviours. Frimley Health saw an increase in staff recommending it as a place to work from 44% to 77% in one year.[21]

Tough love

Few staff would readily associate appraisals and performance management with love. In fact, research shows that even the best employees can go into defensive fight or flight mode when presented with a single score to describe a year's work. Millennials in particular just aren't used to this kind of feedback. In a recent study, 64% reported having felt 'blind-sided' by an appraisal.

On the other hand, a lack of feedback can be just as damaging. Without it, employees can feel anxious and unsure what colleagues think of them. Performance management is important for employers too; unless time is set aside to plan jobs and agree how professional ambitions align with strategic objectives, how else can employers be sure that everyone in the organization is pulling in the same direction?

More and more, performance management is evolving from a once-yearly appraisal into a more continuous two-way conversation, punctuated throughout the year by shorter reviews and discussions. This type of process allows for course correction throughout the year and is more akin to coaching than the brutal 'rank and yank' approach of old. It reframes performance management into talent management—a phrase that probably makes most clinicians feel a bit queasy, but why not? We should think of them as talent. It is also better suited to the kind of collaborative team working we seek to foster in health now. Several high-profile organizations have had success with this method. IBM saw double digit engagement scores growth after introducing continuous performance management, while Adobe's voluntary turnover decreased by 30%.[22]

More and more, I believe we will move away from a focus on individuals to team performance management. This is a far more advanced process in other industries, but we are starting to see something like it in healthcare. Getting It Right First Time is a UK NHS programme that visits medical departments up and down the country and compares performance against 'best in class' and demographic peers.[23] The team can then advise on ways to improve processes and procurement to obtain better clinical and financial results. It is an initiative led and delivered by clinicians—it wouldn't have gone down well if it wasn't.

In other industries, team management has reached an entirely different plane that is only just starting to reveal its potential. Organizational network analysis is a process of mapping working relationships across teams, organizations, and systems. It works on the premise that there is a relationship network running parallel to the rigid organogram in any organization and it is the relationship network that tells you how work really gets done. Some companies are starting to build pictures of these relationship networks by using artificial intelligence to survey workers emails, phone calls, conversations, and movements. They are even starting to correlate this information with performance data on individuals and teams to devise what the most efficient team working looks like.

We may not be as far from this as we think. New Cross Hospital in Wolverhampton, United Kingdom, has recently installed sensors across the hospital. Every worker is fitted with a tracking device (and every patient if they consent). Using this technology, the hospital can track people and processes across the system and work on how to improve patient flow.[24]

When HR meets AI

With so many healthcare employers struggling to meet even the current needs of workforce leadership and management, there will be trouble ahead if organizations do not start preparing now for the world of artificial intelligence.

We have already seen how the rise of the machine will usually replace tasks rather than jobs. This atomization of work is already occurring in many parts of the economy including professional services such as law, engineering, finance, and consulting, leading to new and constantly evolving and adapting organizational forms as old skills become obsolete and new ones are suddenly in demand.

HR professionals will need to get to grips with systems thinking and how they can contribute to end-to-end process redesign as an integral part of their role. The increasing complexity of systems involving both people and machines will increase the risks of a short-term fix in one part of the organization creating serious long-term problems in another. HR teams will also need to provide leadership for constant and overlapping cycles of change management.

From induction to retirement

Workforce retention strategies should focus on retaining professionals at every stage of their career. The first few days, weeks, and months on the job are critical to retention. According to the Robert Wood Johnson Foundation, almost a fifth of US nurses leave the job in their first year. After two years, a third have left.[25]

Preceptorship schemes are part of the Magnet programme, although they have become increasingly popular more generally in the United States and United Kingdom. A cross between induction, mentorship, and internship, the programmes help nurses move from education to employment and improve retention. The programmes usually last between four months and a year and range from providing structured teaching on things like blood transfusion protocols through to social events and networking opportunities for new nurses, with some even putting senior nurses with new recruits on the shop floor to answer questions and give on the job advice.

Research by Capital Nurse, a London-based nurse retention programme, found that the period following preceptorships was also a vulnerable time for retention. In the absence of a clear roadmap for nursing careers, many nurses thought of leaving the profession. The programme introduced a voluntary portfolio that nurses could use to document qualifications and skills, track career progress, and use as a template for career planning with managers and mentors. While such tools are common for doctors this was a big change for London nurses, who said that they had never before had a conversation with anyone at work about their career.[26]

In-house training or reimbursement of training costs is another great retainer. In the United Kingdom, a great deal of further training is subsidized through an educational budget for continuing professional development (CPD). An inquiry by the House of Commons' Health Select Committee into nursing highlighted a 60% cut in the nurses' CPD budget as a major contributor to nurses feeling undervalued and quitting the profession.[27]

Giving professionals the opportunity to move sideways can be just as valuable. At University College London Hospital, nurses considering a move to a different specialty no longer need to move to another employer, because they can ask to do trial shifts before applying for an internal transfer. Clalit in Israel have taken this one step further. As a health maintenance organization (HMO), it is able to offer nurses the ability to transfer not just between specialties but also between workplaces. This means that a nurse who would prefer to work in a fast-paced hospital post when younger and perhaps move into a teaching, research, leadership, or community nursing post later is able to do just that, without switching providers and without the organization incurring a turnover cost.

According to job website Indeed, millennials rate Kaiser Permanente as the third best employer in the United States (it also came top in their ratings for interns). Attractions include allowing staff to create an individual development plan with their manager to help improve their skills and grow their careers, online courses and in-person classes, 'stretch assignments', exploration of new technologies, and the options of participating in leadership training and mentorship programmes.[28] When I met the Kaiser Permanente leadership team in Oakland, California, I was pleased and astonished to learn that many millennial projects had been given to the finance—not HR—team to run, to demonstrate this change was everybody's business.

Holding on to mature talent

Retaining the skills and experience of older workers is going to be a priority as the health workforce ages. According to the most recent National Nursing Workforce Survey in the United States, half of registered nurses were aged 50 or older.[29] Employers will not be able to rely on large numbers of young people entering the labour market. Addressing this is a particular consideration for professionals whose jobs involve a large physical component—nurses, healthcare assistants, surgeons— and all those professionals with irregular hours and night working. This will require better investment in health and well-being throughout the working life and better planning leading up to and throughout older age. This is important for preventing and managing mental illness and musculoskeletal problems, the most common causes of long-term sickness absence.

A number of employers, not just in health, now offer an array of services to keep employees of all ages healthy. Free yoga classes, massages, mindfulness apps, treadmill desks, resilience training—the list is endless. The supermarket Tesco is experimenting with wearable fitness monitors to track employee activity. The problem, according to Theresa Marteau of the behavioural and health research unit at Cambridge University, is an absence of evidence for a lot of wellness schemes.

A 2011 audit of UK trusts showed that half had introduced schemes to encourage cycling or walking to work (such as fitting showers), a third had provided weight management training for staff, and two-thirds had promoted healthy eating in their canteens.[30] Unfortunately, there were few evaluations of impact. In addition, a survey carried out by Rand Europe, the *Financial Times*, and Cambridge estimated that just 28% of employees take up wellness initiatives.[31]

That doesn't mean we shouldn't do any of it, just that it should be guided by evidence. Occupational Health—underappreciated and underused—could have a more central role in healthcare, as it does in other industries. For instance, Steelite in the United Kingdom offers staff access to a monthly on-site occupational health clinic. Employees can either request appointments or are referred following long-term sickness absence or workplace accidents. The occupational health team develops tailored support plans, which might include workplace adjustments, additional equipment or training, and changes to the hours or role.

British Gas introduced a back-care workshop for staff in physically demanding jobs and saw a reduction in back pain-related absence of 43%.[32] But such efforts cannot be made in isolation from other improvements. Otherwise, in the absence of any serious attempt to reduce work stressors, things like free yoga lessons and a mindfulness app start to look piecemeal and tokenistic.

Retirement planning is an area where health can learn a lot from other industries about retaining older workers. A Danish construction company described in a 2016 Chartered Institute of Personnel and Development (CIPD) report holds regular 'senior conversations' with older employees about thoughts and plans for the future.[33] They offer increased flexibility in working hours and task rotation and hold regular conferences to inform older workers of opportunities.

In the Czech Republic, Skoda Auto's Senior Programme comprises an annual agreement negotiated between management and unions focused on enabling the continued employment of people in predominantly manual labour jobs. In Denmark, when employees of bus company Arriva reach 60, they are offered the option to reduce hours under an 80:80:100 or 90:90:100 scheme—under this arrangement, hours and wages are reduced to 80 or 90%, but the employer continues to pay 100% of its pension contribution.

Bringing the flexibility of the gig economy to healthcare

When it comes to improving shift flexibility, e-rostering can offer employees something more akin to the Amazon or Uber gig economy experience, but so often it is used as straightforward digital version of a paper process. Much of it is not new—the idea of self-rostering has been around a long time—although the newest software allows employees to select and swap shifts via a phone app at a time that suits them. But for employers it offers much more. As well as cutting administration and reliance on agency staff, it can help map hospital demand across the week to determine staffing needs, track staffing across the hospital in real time, and allow better deployment of available staff. If the system is linked by cloud with other hospitals in the area, such as through the platform developed by Allocate Software, it can draw on their staff too.

Since initiating Avantas's e-rostering software in 2015, the University of Kansas Hospital has managed to fill 95% of its shifts with core staff, has seen a 65% drop in last-minute work requests, and has halved the time spent by managers scheduling and re-scheduling shifts. Staff turnover fell to its lowest ever rate.[34]

Other industries have gone further. Rather than mapping people to roles, companies are starting to think about mapping skills to tasks, and the technology provided by companies like ProFinda allows them to do it. People upload their skills and work preferences and employers access that to assemble ad hoc teams. It is the gig economy for professionals and it is going to suit millennials, Generation X-ers, and baby boomers alike.

Building connections

For healthcare staff, much of the world of work is still modelled on an approach which may have suited men in the 1950s but is unfit for today's workforce. Making staff feel loved requires a concerted and increasingly tailored approach which builds connections between each person's professional role, personal development, and private life. Health employers are going to have to get on board with this. If they drag their feet, they should not be surprised if staff vote with theirs.

The transformational effects of artificial intelligence should be embraced as an extraordinary opportunity to bring joy to the work of healthcare. Of course, there will be disruption. Roles will constantly change and professional boundaries will be challenged and breached. But the focus on systems thinking and working, plus the sheer intellectual challenge of artificial intelligence can lead to the creation of more engaging, more stimulating, and decidedly more human organizations, with a spirit of shared endeavour and lifelong learning. One day, we might move from a world where we are what we do, to a world where we do what we are.

Chapter 12

Women's work? Altogether now

Women make up a large and increasing proportion of the global healthcare workforce. As an industry, healthcare seems to welcome more women than most, typically ranking alongside sectors such as education and childcare in female participation rates. Nursing and clerical roles within the sector have been predominately female for some time, so much of the recent growth has been driven by a steady rise in the number of women doctors. This worldwide phenomenon, which began in the 1970s, is dubbed the 'feminization of medicine'.

Yet despite such strong female representation in the health workforce there are wide inequalities between men and women within it. Men still earn more and dominate leadership positions. Women are more likely to experience discrimination and harassment at work and are more likely to tame ambitions, cut hours, or drop out of the labour force after having children. In the face of acute workforce shortages, efforts to tackle these issues to attract, engage, and retain female staff will become increasingly important to both employers and governments.

So too will be the need to focus on structural and cultural barriers preventing workers in predominantly female roles, such as nursing, take on greater professional responsibility—crucial if health systems are to move towards new and more productive models of care.

Healthcare may simultaneously have to find ways to make caring jobs more attractive to men, as automation erodes traditionally male manual jobs and countries move towards more service-led economies, with healthcare jobs front and centre.

Pursuing gender equality is a moral necessity, and as one of the UN's 17 Sustainability and Development Goals it is recognized as one of the foundations for a prosperous and peaceful society. It is also what younger generations of both sexes increasingly want and expect. Happily there is also an overwhelming business case for gender equity in the workplace—countries and companies with greater equity are better off for it.

The facts

The International Labour Organization (ILO) estimates around 70% of workers in health and social care globally are women. This compares with an average participation figure for women across all sectors of about 40%.[1] High-income countries have the highest proportion of women at 77%, while low- and lower-middle-income countries have the lowest, at around 47%. This trend is consistent across regions. Even in the Arab states, where women make up just 16% of the workforce, they make up 38% of the health and social care staff. Clearly, as Figure 12.1 illustrates,

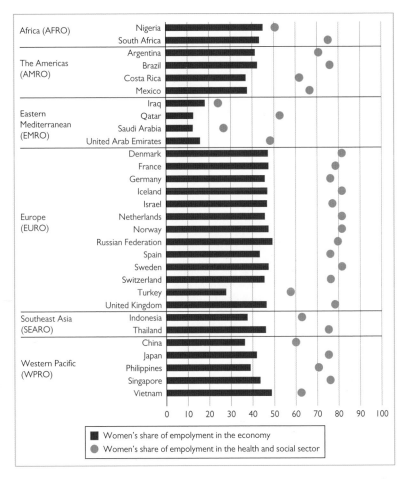

Fig. 12.1 Women's share of employment in the health and social sector versus total employment (%), by World Health Organization (WHO) region, average values for the period 2005–2014.

Reproduced with permission from Buchan, J. et al. (Eds). Health Employment and Economic Growth: An Evidence Base. Geneva, Switzerland: World Health Organization. Copyright © 2017 WHO.

health and social care work is an important source of employment for women across the world.

Within healthcare, further themes emerge around gender. Nursing has the highest proportion of women in a profession no matter where you go. In Organisation for Economic Co-operation and Development (OECD) countries, around 90–95% of nurses are women. In China and Iceland, that figure is closer to 99%. Saudi Arabia has the lowest rate, but it is still 77%.[2]

Within medicine, the proportion of female doctors varies more widely. The nation with the highest rate is Russia, followed swiftly by other mainly Eastern European states—Latvia, Estonia, Slovenia, Finland, Slovak Republic, Poland, Hungary, and Czech Republic.[3] This is a legacy from the 1950s and the Soviet era when medicine was deprofessionalized. Medical societies were abolished, physicians became state employees, and Russian doctors lost control of their profession. At the same time, women were encouraged to apply and medicine simultaneously lost status and became one of the poorest paid Eastern bloc professions. Since then, women have comprised upwards of about 70–75% of the physician workforce in Russia and surrounding states.[4]

After Russia and the Eastern European states come Scandinavia and Europe. The United States has a fairly low share of female doctors—just 34%. South Korea and Japan have the lowest share of female physicians of the OECD countries—22% and 20%.[5]

The low proportion of female doctors in Japan is partly down to the legacy of recruiting few women into medical school. The recent revelation that Tokyo Medical University—one of Japan's most prestigious medical schools—had manipulated entrance examination results for at least a decade to ensure fewer women became medical students exposes the endemic discrimination against women in the Japanese medical workforce. The fact that this scandal happened at a university which had been given extra government money specifically to increase the number of female medical students only adds to the insult.

Those women in Japan who do qualify face tremendous difficulties in staying there. Just nine years after graduation, 75% of those female physicians are no longer in employment, primarily because of childcare responsibilities.[6] This is typical for working women in Japan, although many do go back to work after taking time off to have children.

The feminization of medicine will see rates of female participation rise across the world. Women now make up almost a third of new doctors in Japan and around half of new doctors in the United Kingdom, Canada, United States, Australia, and Europe. Low- and middle-income countries are experiencing the same effect. China and India now have rough gender parity in medical school graduates, as do Mexico and Ecuador, for example.

Specialisms

Women tend to specialize in the same areas of medicine worldwide. Family medicine, paediatrics, and obstetrics and gynaecology are common, and this preference has changed little over time even as the proportion of women in medicine has increased (see Fig. 12.2).

For example, in 1980 around 12% of medical graduates in the United States were women. They made up about 56% of paediatricians, 54% of gynaecologists, 46% of dermatologists, and 45% of endocrinologists. Orthopaedics was the least popular choice, with just 4% women.

Their choices (and the cohorts after them) shaped the current distribution of specialties. Fast-forward 35 years to 2015 and almost half of medical graduates are

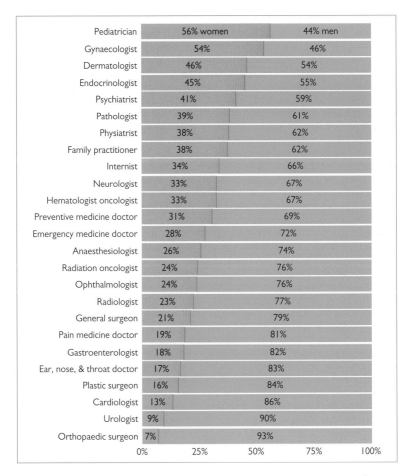

Fig. 12.2 Not all specialties are (gender) equal: gender breakdown of common doctor specialties.
Reproduced with permission from Levy, H. How the gender gap is shifting in medicine, by specialty.
Amino Blog, 14 Sept 2016. Copyright © 2016 Amino. Available at https://amino.com/blog/
how-the-gender-gap-is-shifting-in-medicine-medical-specialties-by-gender/

women, but the top choices are the same. If anything, the proportion of women
going into them had increased; 83% of new gynaecologists were now women, 77%
of endocrinologists, 71% of paediatricians, and 66% of dermatologists. Orthopaedic
surgery was still the least popular specialty for women, at 15%.[7]

There is a lot of debate about what drives these choices—whether it is innate preference, cultural expectations, the ability to combine it with family life, a lack of female
role models, or macho culture in other specialties. It is certainly true that in studies
of female doctors in the United Kingdom, women report placing more emphasis on

balancing the demands of professional and personal lives when choosing a specialty. In Ecuador, a 2016 study found that gendered norms regarding women's primary role in childrearing had a significant effect on specialty choice.[8]

Women clinicians—both doctors and nurses—tend to work fewer hours. In the United States, the 2016 Medscape Female Physician Compensation Report showed that 40% of male physicians spent 46 hours or more per week with patients compared with just 26% of women.[9] This discrepancy is generally considered to result from the time women dedicate to domestic and childrearing duties. A recent *Journal of the American Medical Association (JAMA)* article looking at the working patterns of dual-physician households in the United States seems to support this. Women doctors tended to work 11 fewer hours a week after having children. Men's hours, however, did not change.[10]

The effects of part-time working are obviously most pronounced in those specialties where women dominate. In the United Kingdom, for example, about 42% of female GPs work part-time compared with about 18% of male GPs, whereas in hospital about 24% of female doctors work part-time compared with 8% of men.[11] Men in hospital specialties are more likely to work in private practice in their spare time, whereas women are more likely to use that time to care for their families.

However, it is important not to assume that all changes to women's work hours are because of childcare. A 2016 King's Fund report on pressures in general practice found the most commonly cited reason for part-time working among both men and women was not family commitments but intensity of the working day. Both male and female GPs were increasingly inclined to work around three days in a GP patient-facing role and combining it with something else such as medical education or other clinical NHS work as part of a portfolio career.[12]

The aggregate figures hide another trend. Younger doctors of both sexes—millennials—are working fewer hours in patient-facing general practice. In 2017, UK GP workforce statistics showed that the average number of hours worked by GPs had fallen 10%.[13] A 2017 Dutch study showed that GPs in their 50s worked the highest number of hours, followed by those in their 60s, with the lowest number of hours worked by those under 40, the effect of shorter hours worked by both male and female GPs.[14]

Men in charge

A consistent trend across continents is that female clinicians occupy fewer leadership positions. This spans clinical leadership, academia, professional bodies, and hospital or practice boards. Amazingly this even applies to nursing, where more men occupy leadership positions despite upwards of 90% of the world's nurses being women.

An Association of American Medical Colleges' report from 2014 describes the 'leaky pipeline' in US academic medicine. While making up about 47% of medical school graduates, women make up just 38% of faculty staff, 21% of full professors, and 16% of deans.[15] A 2015 Christmas issue of the *British Medical Journal (BMJ)* published a tongue-in-cheek study from the University of Pennsylvania showing that while just 13% of department leaders at top academic medical institutions in the United States were female, 20% were men with moustaches.[16] Some—but by no means all—of this discrepancy is down to female physicians being less likely to work full time or because they engage in activities not typically associated with academic productivity (such as teaching or patient care).

The culture that necessitated the #MeToo movement extends to health academia. A 2017 study of US academics found 30% of female physician-scientists experienced sexual harassment compared with 4% of their male counterparts, and while 66% of women said they had experienced gender bias in their academic environment, only 10% of men reported the same.[17]

Of all leadership positions, women are probably least represented at the highest ranks of hospitals. A 2015 US Medscape study of women physician leaders found that while 35% reported their leadership position as medical director, just 3% identified themselves as chief executive and the same proportion as chief medical officer.

Women are probably best represented in clinical leadership positions but even here they face setbacks. In a survey of over 1,300 Japanese obstetricians, a significantly higher proportion of men reported handling deliveries and performing surgeries.[18] Women described 'giving up' these procedures earlier than their male counterparts, citing childcare responsibilities resulting in fewer working hours, fewer night duties, and lower income.

Confidence gap

Other studies point to an ingrained 'confidence gap' between men and women, which can be demonstrated from the early stages of training. A UK study of trainee trauma and orthopaedic surgeons found that when self-rating for appraisal, 58% of male trainees considered themselves outstanding in at least one aspect of work, compared with just 14% of women. Trainers claimed 57% of female trainees needed more confidence, compared with just 8% of men.

Last, and by no means least, women are paid less than men. According to a survey of 65,000 US doctors by social networking platform Doximity, women doctors earned an average 28% less than their male counterparts in 2017, which amounted to $105,000 a year.[19] Part of this discrepancy can be ascribed to differences in leadership positions, specialty choice, and part-time working—but again, not all. The gender pay gap also varies by specialty—it is greatest in male-dominated specialties—and by region—for example, South Carolina has a gap of 37%.

Pay transparency is thought to reduce gender pay differentials but even in the United Kingdom, where national pay scales for NHS doctors are public, there are discrepancies. A recent BBC investigation into consultant pay found an average gender salary gap of £14,000, with most of this difference attributed to clinical award bonuses and overtime. Intriguingly, women were just as likely to receive a clinical award bonus if they applied (both men and women had success rates of 26%) but women were far less likely to do so. This meant that women accounted for just 21% of the awards despite representing 35% of the consultants.[20]

So those are the facts. How are we to interpret them? The feminization of medicine has caused a great deal of handwringing in recent years. Even in Japan, the OECD country with the lowest share of female doctors, academics point to rota gaps and ask whether the feminization of medicine is making the health workforce crisis worse.[21]

This argument gained traction in the United Kingdom a few years back when a professor of surgery from the famous Royal Marsden cancer hospital in London wrote an opinion piece for a national newspaper decrying the feminization of medicine. His objection was that 'most female doctors end up working part-time—usually in general practice—and then retire early. As a result, it is necessary to train two female doctors so they can cover the same amount of work as one full-time colleague. Given that the cost of training a doctor is at least £500,000, are taxpayers getting the best return on their investment?'.

To which the simple answer is: yes. Investment in the education of women has driven higher rates of female participation and is a rich source of global economic growth. I do not believe, as the professor does, that this increase in female participation should be limited to lower skilled and lower paid jobs, however more productive he thinks that set-up might be. In fact, since most higher education is subsidized to some extent in the United Kingdom, this kind of logic would take us into the dystopian territory of evaluating jobs to determine the ones where women represent a good return on investment and the ones in which they do not. I have yet to see an article about the poor return on investment from training a 90% female nursing workforce.

This takes us to the heart of what this argument is really about—not money, but misogyny. It's the fact that in his opinion there is men's work and women's work and never the twain shall meet (unless you are prepared to remain childless or employ a full-time nanny). Women already make up 70% of the healthcare workforce. We should be thinking of ways to retain them, not repel them.

Parenthood and work

The evidence is that family-friendly working, rather than being part of the problem, is part of the solution. Without it, we risk losing parents from the workforce. It needs to be easier to combine parenthood and work and it should be possible for men and women to share that burden equally if they choose. That means shared parental leave, reintegrating parents back into the workforce after prolonged periods of absence, flexible work schedules, and practical childcare support.

Unfortunately, according to the World Bank, only half the economies it examined have paternity leave and less than a third offer shared parental leave.[22] Even in countries where such laws exist it can take time for attitudes to change. In Sweden, the first country to introduce shared parental leave, uptake by men was low until a one month leave 'use it or lose it' clause was introduced for dads.

The absence of legislation does not prevent workplaces from introducing such measures. In the United States, a country with notoriously miserly maternity leave legislation, Fortune 500 companies have been competing to attract and retain female talent with generous parental leave benefits. The problem is that generally only a few high-earning staff are entitled to them.

Easing clinicians back into old jobs is important. Going back to any form of job can be daunting, but lost confidence and competence can be a major barrier for those returning to fast-paced and high stakes clinical practice. In recognition of this, the London School of Paediatrics runs a free course on returning to acute clinical practice, to teach updated guidelines, simulate paediatric emergencies, and help parents build informal networks. Paid returner schemes for GPs and nurses have been successful in the United Kingdom for those looking to return after longer periods away.

Far from being the cause of the workforce crisis, flexible working helps retain parents. This is where ideas such as e-rostering and self-rostering come into their own. According to the Kaiser Family Foundation in the United States, around 4 in 10 working mothers in healthcare say they miss work when a sick child needs to stay at home (compared with just 3% of men), and lack of flexibility is the most common reason nurses returning to the workforce give for having left in the first place.[23] Self-rostering allows parents or carers to schedule work around caring responsibilities, and some e-rosters permit staff to swap shifts at short notice.

Flexible, family-friendly working doesn't just mean offering the opportunity to work part-time. It is also about other family friendly practices such as permission to work from home when appropriate, paid parental leave, restricting meetings to office (and childcare-friendly) hours, and having a predictable work schedule to arrange childcare around, which means getting clinical rotas well in advance and ensuring shifts finish on time.

It also means practical support with childcare, whether cost, convenience, or both. Cost, it turns out, is probably the biggest factor for most. A survey of UK working mothers by online chat forum Mumsnet and the Resolution Foundation think tank found 67% of mothers in work and 64% of those not working said the high cost of childcare is a barrier to taking on more employment. Four out of ten of the women identified childcare costs as the single biggest obstacle to taking on more work.[24] The ILO found that in countries where governments support childcare, such as through funding free childcare hours, women are much more likely to be employed.

Employers can also help with convenience. Onsite childcare facilities are a relatively common example, but not common enough. The Brigham and Women's Hospital in Boston goes one step further and offers all workers a reduced rate for six days of emergency childcare at home plus access to a backup childcare centre that can be activated with as little as two hours' notice.

Every healthcare provider of reasonable size should provide a creche for the children of staff. It is the right thing to do and it would improve retention, cut absenteeism, and make a statement about gender equality. The US-based Parenting in the Workplace Institute has found that the biggest benefits to businesses for providing access to nursery facilities are retention and recruitment.

As well as making it equally possible to work in health, we also need to think about making it equally rewarding, both in comparison with men and with other sectors of employment. That means addressing fair pay, opportunities for career progression, and the workplace experience.

This encompasses a lot, but there are a few obvious things with which employers can start. For example, the American Medical Women's Association believe greater pay transparency would make a big difference to narrowing the gender pay gap in medicine. Other ideas include better access to mentors and a commitment to open and fair nominations for leadership positions.

Unleashing the potential of nurses

Finally, I need to say something about gender bias and the effect it has had in limiting the predominantly female profession of nursing.

For decades, nurses have been taking on roles and responsibilities once thought to be the preserve of physicians. There are nurses in Mozambique performing c-sections, nurses in South Africa diagnosing and treating HIV, and nurse anaesthesiologists in the United States. This trend could grow as machine learning and medical technology develop, affording health systems the opportunity to move towards care models that are more productive, faster to scale, and cheaper.

Consistently, however, efforts to grant nurses even strongly evidence-based skills such as prescribing rights are thwarted. Take the example of nurse practitioners in the United States. Despite 50 years of evidence to support the safety and effectiveness of nurse practitioners delivering primary care services, wide variations in the regulation of nurses persist between states, restricting nurse practitioners from carrying out the work they have been trained to do. Gender is not the only reason, but it is part of it.

A study comparing nursing regulations in states that ratified the Equal Rights Amendment to the US Constitution (which has still not been approved more than 40 years after Congress passed it) with regulations in states that opposed the amendment found that more than half of supportive states gave nurse practitioners full practice authority compared with only a fifth of those that did not support it.[25]

The perception of nursing as a predominantly female profession may be holding it back in other ways too—it could be limiting its potential for growth. According to the Bureau of Labor Statistics, the two jobs predicted to decline most quickly from 2014 to 2024 in the United States are 98% male—locomotive firers (predicted to fall 70%) and vehicle electronics installers and repairers (50%).[26] Yet despite the loss of American blue-collar jobs to robots or production lines in China and Mexico, men are not taking up new roles in the growing sector of 'pink-collar jobs' like healthcare. While such jobs are often less well paid than blue-collar ones, the evidence suggests one of the biggest issues is the stigma that still surrounds men taking caring roles. Harvard economist Lawrence Kratz calls it an 'identity mismatch' rather than a 'skills mismatch', reflecting the struggle of many men in manual jobs to adapt to the changing economy which drove, at least in part, the nature of political discourse during the American election of 2016.

Elevating the status and profile of nursing is an important step in overcoming these biases and allowing health systems to move towards innovative and more productive models of care—something which the international campaign Nursing Now, in conjunction with the World Health Organization and International Council of Nurses, is trying to do. This means more nurses in leadership positions, better terms and working conditions, and expanded scopes of practice to permit greater nursing career progression.

We can't miss out on talent

In a sector so overwhelmingly female, the inequalities that persist between men and women in terms of their status, pay, and working lives are disturbing. As industries around us get their own house in order on these issues, healthcare risks being left behind, missing out on a wealth of female talent, and stunting its own growth because of stereotyped, outdated attitudes to gender. With multiple opportunities for skilled work, healthcare has the potential to drive gender parity worldwide. Let's be a leader, not a laggard.

Chapter 13

Australia—golden soil and wealth for toil

I first visited and worked in Australia 28 years ago. I was mesmerized by its vastness and beauty. It is incredible to think that ever since my first visit, Australia has set a new world record by enjoying 27 consecutive years of economic growth. It is on the right side of the world at just the right time in history, as Asia rises. It consistently ranks highly in the Organisation for Economic Co-operation and Development (OECD) Better Life Index[1] which looks at the level of well-being in society. Indeed, the title of this chapter takes some of the lyrics out of the Australian national anthem, Advance Australia Fair. Its healthcare staff are well paid and looked after and clinical facilities are often good, but Australia's workforce challenges are shaped by the vastness of its land and the enduring inequalities in health outcomes of its Aboriginal and Torres Strait Islander people.

Good pay, good life

Among overseas doctors coming to Australia, many thousands of Europeans have been attracted by better pay, shorter hours, and the impression of more manageable jobs with less bureaucracy. The decision in 2016 to tighten visa rules for foreign doctors was in part driven by a surge in applications from junior doctors in the United Kingdom demoralized by their dispute with the government over pay and conditions.[2]

According to 2016 data from Medic Footprints, Australia was second only to the Netherlands in doctors' salaries. Consultants typically earn AU$175–350,000 (US$127–254,000, £100–200,000) while GPs earn around AU$200–350,000 (US$145–254,000, £114–200,000), and registrars AU$75–110,000 (US$54–80,000, £43–63,000).[3]

As well as the pay, posts from UK expatriates in blogs and doctors' forums often refer to a good work-life balance. Hospital doctors talk about manageable hours in well-staffed, well-equipped facilities, and they are paid overtime when they work more than 38 hours and for weekends and night shifts. Funding is also available to support GPs providing after-hours cover. The Australian Medical Association (AMA) says that that while there has been a big reduction in the number of doctors exposed to excessive working hours since the 1990s, one in two are still working rosters that put them at significant risk of fatigue.[4]

UK doctors who emigrate there often say they feel more valued by their employer. Training opportunities and quality are attractive. Respected, well paid, well resourced, a good work-life balance, and all in an extraordinary country—no wonder

Australia has become a magnet for international medical talent. As Commonwealth Fund data reveals, GPs in Australia are among the least stressed (although that is a low benchmark—see Fig. 13.1).

It is a similar story for nurses. Australian nurses are among the highest paid in the world. A registered nurse or midwife would expect to start on around AU$60,000 (US$43,000, £34,000) and reach a maximum of around AU$85,000 (US$62,000, £48,000). As well as attractive pay and feeling valued, a typical nurse in a public hospital may well be looking after four patients; hospitals in England struggle to keep it to eight.[5]

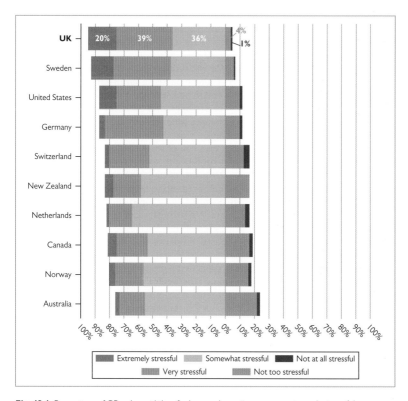

Fig. 13.1 Percentage of GPs who said they find general practice very or extremely stressful.

Reproduced with permission from Gershlick, B. et al. A sustainable workforce—the lifeblood of the NHS and social care. Election briefing May 2017. Copyright © The Health Foundation. Available at www.health.org.uk/publication/election-briefing-sustainable-workforce

The challenge of remote areas

The country is in the unusual position of simultaneously having both a shortage and an oversupply of medical graduates. The problem arises because, despite a surge in graduate numbers, Australia struggles to get doctors to work in rural and remote areas, home to roughly a fifth of the country's 25 million people. Among Australian medical students, working in rural medicine is seen as neither prestigious nor an attractive lifestyle (see Fig. 13.2).

This means the country remains heavily reliant on doctors trained overseas, especially GPs, and is far more dependent on overseas recruitment than most OECD countries. So medical graduates risk being unable to find a job they want while vacancies in rural and remote areas go unfilled. International medical graduates now make up more than 40% of the rural medical workforce. There are similar rural shortages in nursing and allied health professionals.

The AMA has called for at least one-third of all new medical students to be drawn from rural backgrounds and for medical students to be required to do at least one year of training in rural and remote areas.[6]

Building a sustainable rural workforce will require more than just increasing the number of in-country appointments. Training needs to ensure they have the right skills to work in rural areas. Facilities need to be improved. Professional support and education, including relief by locums, need to upgraded. Salaries need to be competitive. Importantly, partners and children need support such as housing subsidies and employment and education opportunities.

The AMA cites the closure of more than half of small rural maternity units in the last 20 years as evidence of decline in rural health services—driven in part by the difficulty of balancing ease of access with quality of care. The need for improvements is pressing, with life expectancy in remote areas up to seven years lower than cities, and higher rates of coronary heart disease, COPD, cancer, and suicide.

The Australian Institute of Health and Welfare estimates there are 437 full-time equivalent doctors per 100,000 population in major cities, compared with 272 in rural areas and 264 in the remotest parts of the country. Rural GPs tend to work substantially longer hours.[7]

The federal government has appointed its first national rural health commissioner. He has been promoting the Rural Junior Doctor Training Innovation Fund, which gives junior doctors experience in rural general practice in addition to their hospital-based rotations.[8] The General Practice Rural Incentives Program provides incentives for doctors to work in rural and remote areas.[9]

The Queensland Rural Generalist Pathway is an example of how the states and territories are trying to attract medical talent to sparsely populated areas. It promises strong personal, professional, and administrative support, rapid progress up pay scales, and no lock-in period. Trainees will gain experience in paediatrics, anaesthetics, obstetrics, and gynaecology. It appeals to the adventurous, and can lead to postings such as international aid work and expeditionary medicine. But the connection with aid work gives an indication of how demanding the role of rural generalist can be, requiring personal resilience and professional self-reliance. The Rural Generalist Pathway is now being adopted nationally.[10]

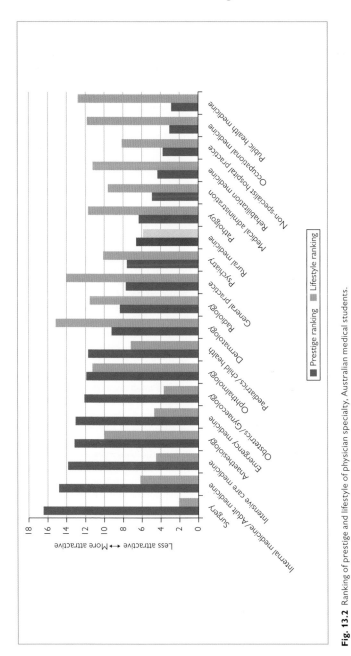

Fig. 13.2 Ranking of prestige and lifestyle of physician specialty, Australian medical students.
Reproduced with permission from Buchan, J., et al. (Eds). Health Employment and Economic Growth: An Evidence Base. Geneva, Switzerland: World Health Organization. Copyright © 2017 WHO.

Building the size and skills of the nursing workforce

There is a looming shortage of nurses and midwives. In 2014 the Department of Health forecast a national shortage of around 123,000 nurses by 2030. This compares with a total workforce in 2015 of 307,000.

Since then improved retention rates as the economy slows means predictions of the shortfall are coming down sharply, but it will not come close to being eliminated. The age of the workforce is one factor driving the shortage, with a quarter of registered nurses aged 55 and over. As always, the government hopes that immigration will make up the shortfall, with nursing set remain on the Skilled Occupation List which prioritizes work visas. However, the number of nurses holding skilled visas has dropped from a recent peak of around 5,000 in 2013 to nearer 2,000.

Unified regulation

The Council of Australian Governments' (COAG) Health Council is examining recommendations for overhauling the accreditation systems for healthcare professionals, possibly by bringing them together under a single cross-professions board. The review has found that the current National Registration and Accreditation Scheme has multiple overlapping regulators, including 14 accreditation authorities and many other bodies having accreditation functions.[11]

The AMA is resisting, claiming some of the proposals could allow the government to take drastic action such as 'import 20,000 doctors from West Africa . . . Or, with the stroke of a pen, governments can try to fix their problems by having nurses do more or other health workers act outside their scope'.[12] But building a single register has much to recommend it, including clearer accountability to the public and the creation of national datasets to support the modelling of workforce needs.

The AMA has opposed the development of independent nurse practitioners, one of the important reforms of recent years. A statement in 2015 said general practice nurses should not work independently of GPs, should not refer patients to specialists, should not order pathology, and should not issue repeat prescriptions. Feedback from nurses included accusations that the statement was myopic, inaccurate, outdated, arrogant, and patronizing. The issue of autonomous working is particularly important in remote areas where the nearest doctor could be hundreds of miles away. More recently, independent nurse practitioners are gradually becoming more accepted by doctors as part of the solution to rural workforce shortages. As we know, it works perfectly well in other parts of the world.

Advanced practice roles are being explored across a number of Australian jurisdictions in response to the need to drive more efficient and effective workforce models. There has been a particular focus on advanced practice nursing and allied health roles. Nationally the Nursing and Midwifery Board of Australia is promoting advanced nursing roles such as endoscopy and cystoscopy. The state of Victoria is a leading exponent of advanced practice roles, where they are supporting major projects in disciplines such as physiotherapy, pharmacy, exercise physiology, and continence. For example, advance physiotherapy roles are being used to support arthroplasty clinics, emergency departments, chronic disease rehabilitation, neuro-surgery outpatient clinics, and women's health programmes. Victoria claims that using advanced practice physiotherapists in post-arthroplasty reviews cut the cost of each appointment by 41% while maintaining care quality.[13]

The state's reforms are being driven by the sector-led Health Workforce Reform Implementation Taskforce, set up six years ago. It aims to get allied health professionals and advanced practice roles into the mainstream of care provision, with an emphasis on community provision and care of older people.

Mental health

Australia provides one of the most impressive mental health services I have encountered, but even here, rural areas lose out heavily. Cities have four times the number of psychiatrists per 100,000 people, four times the psychologists, and three times the nurses compared with the most remote areas. Staff in remote areas work longer hours.

Around 800 non-governmental organizations play a significant role in mental health provision, providing around 12,000 doctors, nurses, and psychologists compared with a total of around 50,000. Many of these organizations are community led.[14]

National fragmentation

The biggest obstacle to improving workforce planning and modernizing care provision to meet changing needs is the fragmentation of control and funding across the healthcare system. Broadly speaking, the federal authorities run primary care while the states run the hospitals. The funding streams are separate, and employment relationships are complicated by many doctors having distinct arrangements from all the other healthcare staff. There is both public and private provision—and the public sector picks up most of the bill for training.

According to Crettenden et al., previous attempts at developing a comprehensive workforce plan had been undermined by a silo approach focused on individual specialisms and the failure to connect the health system with higher education.

After years of discussions about the best way for the federal government, state governments and territories to plan the health workforce, in 2008 COAG finally agreed that a national, coordinated approach to health workforce reform was needed.[15]

Health Workforce Australia was established as the national agency to progress health workforce reform. It developed Australia's first major, long-term national workforce projections for doctors, nurses, and midwives over a planning horizon to 2025 (called Health Workforce 2025), which provided a national platform for developing policies to help ensure Australia's health workforce met the community's needs.

But Health Workforce Australia's planning horizon proved longer than its lifespan. The government shut it in 2014, leaving the states and territories to take the lead on the workforce planning. When migration policy is such an important part of workforce policy, it is questionable whether this can be managed effectively without greater federal oversight. There is a national Health Workforce Planning Committee, but its impact remains to be seen.

Aboriginal and Torres Strait Islander health workers

While there have certainly been significant improvements in recent years in health services and outcomes for indigenous Australians, serious inequalities persist. Average life expectancy for these communities is 10 years shorter than the rest of the population.[16]

Aboriginal and Torres Strait Islander people make up around 3% of the population but account for less than 1% of the healthcare workforce. They are overwhelmingly involved in providing services for their own communities after completing training specifically aimed at the needs of indigenous people, and are known as Aboriginal and Torres Strait Islander Health Practitioners. There is wide variation across the country in terms of their roles, training, employment conditions, and how they interact with the other members of the health system.

Aboriginal and Torres Strait Islander Health Practitioners are particularly involved in primary care, such as clinical assessments, monitoring, and health promotion. Staff are employed in programmes such as Aboriginal Community Controlled Health Services and Aboriginal Medical Service.[17]

One of the barriers to attracting more Aboriginal and Torres Strait Islander people into the healthcare workforce and expanding their role has been arguments over professional recognition for the role of Aboriginal and Torres Strait Islander Health Practitioners, including how the registration system works and how professional qualifications compare with other parts of the system. A measure of how far there is to go in developing the potential of the Aboriginal and Torres Strait Islander healthcare workforce is the fact that the number educated to degree level is still just a few hundred.

Telehealth

For a country which struggles to get medical services into isolated areas, the potential of telehealth is obvious, and its advance is being helped by funding changes introduced in 2011 to promote its use and federal work to improve the reach of the broadband system. Early successes include trials with mental health consultations in rural and remote areas. However, a 2016 review found the integration of telehealth was slow and fragmented, with many pilot programmes not developing into sustained services.[18]

Queensland and Western Australia are leading the way. Queensland Health is running more than 2,000 telehealth systems, including many video consultation facilities, while in Western Australia the Emergency Telehealth Service supports clinical staff in emergency departments, as well as linking patients to Perth-based specialists.[19]

Conclusion

The vast and remote nature of much of this wonderful country means providing comprehensive care will always be a challenge, so it needs to do even more to attract home-grown talent to work in its most inaccessible areas. It also needs to further leverage its world-leading position (along with Canada) in telehealth and telecare.

The best example I have seen, which I referred to in Chapter 5 and is genuinely world-class, is Silver Chain, the largest provider of in-home health and aged care in Perth and Western Australia. I first saw their services demonstrated at one of our global health conferences in Hong Kong, roughly 3,750 miles away from this beautiful state. They have pioneered both the concept and practice of the 'holoporter' where a doctor appears in the form of a hologram inside the patient's own home. The patient is accompanied by the nurse, who have super-extended roles, but have the holographic back-up of the doctor who appears in front of both the patient and nurse through a visor. It looks futuristic—and it is. But it is also extremely comforting and reassuring for patients who wish to stay at home for as long as possible. Silver Chain has been going for over 100 years, but they do not let traditions stand in the way of innovation and progress.

Finally, the financial rewards, status, and working environment accorded to Australian healthcare staff is a model for others to follow. It is not just the money— manageable hours, proportionate bureaucracy, and a sense of being valued allows clinicians to focus on getting to the top of their game. But with these privileges should come a greater accountability to change some rather traditional role and task demarcations which, happily and satisfactorily, have been settled years ago in other countries. Australians don't like coming second; it's time to step up.

Chapter 14

The United Kingdom—the age of austerity

Uniquely, the British chose to illustrate all that is good with our country by show-casing the National Health Service (NHS) at the opening of the London Olympics in 2012. In the United Kingdom, the NHS is considered the proudest achievement of modern society and continues to enjoy satisfaction ratings higher than the Royal Family. I have never worked in another country where the values of its health service are so inextricably linked with its national consciousness and character (although Costa Rica and Canada might take silver and bronze medals).

Yet the United Kingdom is going through tectonic challenges and changes as we face Brexit and find our new place in the world order. Naturally, this affects the NHS and the people who work for it. As we debate what our national identity means, it is vital we remember why the NHS makes us so proud and the values it upholds because, in an increasingly fractured and polarized United Kingdom, it reminds us of what keeps us together. While we have four similar yet distinct health systems across England, Scotland, Wales, and Northern Ireland, the rest of this chapter concentrates solely on the English NHS.

Riding high

Ten years ago, the NHS was riding high. At the end of the financial year 2009–2010, the NHS had never, in its history, enjoyed higher ratings for public, patient, and staff satisfaction (see Fig. 14.1). Waiting lists were low, quality was improving, the NHS was in healthy financial balance, and sustained improvements had been made to major clinical outcomes for cancer, stroke, and heart disease. There was a decent government strategy to reduce health inequalities through a variety of measures which included the introduction of the minimum wage, Sure Start for children in their early years, investment in local government, and excellent job creation across the United Kingdom. Health inequalities were narrowing while life expectancy was increasing.

This was no accident. A decade before, during the winter of 1999, the health service had been brought to its knees through a surge in patient demand and inadequate capacity. Hospitals were full, discharges were delayed, and ambulances waited. Primary care was overrun and mental health services were overstretched. Then, as a chief operating officer of University Hospitals Birmingham (UHB), I remember, just before Christmas, walking around each ward and counting (the information systems didn't exist) nearly 300 patients—around a quarter of our beds—unable to leave because they could not find a care home place or get social care support. Our hospitals were

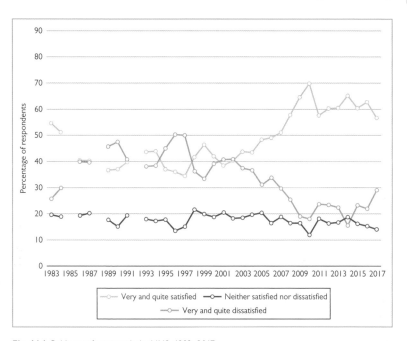

Fig. 14.1 Public satisfaction with the NHS, 1983–2017.

Reproduced with permission from King's Fund and Nuffield Trust analysis of NatCen Social Research's BSA survey data. Copyright © 2018 The Nuffield Trust and The King's Fund.

grinding to a halt. The government listened to staff, patients, and the public, and decided to bring health investment up to European levels.

The NHS Plan was developed and I was a member of the Professions Modernisation Action Team that recommended a significant increase in the workforce and its pay. The NHS Plan also invested heavily in new infrastructure (hospitals, primary care centres, and equipment) and targeted improvements in waiting times and cancer, stroke, and cardiac outcomes, where performance was much worse than the European average. New management and clinical improvement techniques were introduced at scale through the Modernisation Agency and a robust national performance management system was put into place. High performing and successful hospitals were given more freedom and as chief executive of University Hospitals Birmingham I was able to 'design and sign' the largest single new hospital (the Queen Elizabeth Hospital) in the history of the NHS and make our organization 'self-governing' with new freedoms to serve our local communities, patients, and staff.

Later that decade, in a sign of the growing self-confidence of the NHS, the first NHS Constitution was introduced around its sixtieth birthday and the government published High Quality Care for All, a staff-led document mapping out the next stage of the service's development. I was proud to be a member of the NHS Management Board that introduced both. The constitution set out rights for patients, the public, and staff, and articulated the responsibilities that patients, the public, and staff owe to one another. As importantly and for the first time, it explicitly crystallized the values which the NHS held dear. I remember being involved in some sensitive discussions with ministers at the time but the intention was always clear: to openly commit to values and standards that could be measured and judged by future generations.

Crash

And then the global financial crisis happened. The outgoing Labour government took action to avoid a second Great Depression, but public finances started to feel the pinch. The Conservative and Liberal Democrat Coalition government of 2010–2015 took decisive action to reduce the national burden of debt and this was continued by Conservative governments from 2015 onwards. Britain's longest and deepest recession of the post-war era ushered in an age of austerity for the NHS with consequences for patients and staff alike. Since 2009–2010, NHS funding has grown in real terms by 1.1% to 2014–2015 and by 2.3% onwards. This compares with historic growth, from the inception of the NHS in 1948, of 3.7%.[1]

Compared with other public services such as social care and public health, which have been cut sharply, the NHS has actually fared quite well, continuing to take an increasing chunk of the national economy along with a larger proportion of government spending (up from 23% in 1999–2000 to 30% in 2016–2017).[2] But rising demand from a growing and ageing population has quickly absorbed the meagre funding increases while increasing patient complexity has left staff to cope with sharply growing workloads.

The NHS cannot hide from the consequences. By the end of 2017–2018, the service missed most of the standards set out in the constitution. As Sir Chris Ham, former chief executive of the King's Fund, says: 'The NHS has not met the standard that 95% of patients should be seen within four hours in A&E since July 2015. The number of people on waiting lists for elective treatment is now more than 4 million, and the standard that 92% of patients should start treatment within 18 weeks of referral has not been achieved since February 2016. The standard that 85% of patients should begin definitive treatment for cancer within 62 days of referral was last achieved in quarter three of 2013/14.'[3] Behind every one of these numbers and statistics is a human being waiting for care and treatment.

The hospital regulator, NHS Improvement, announced in September 2018 that the underlying deficit for NHS providers had reached an historic high of £4.3 billion. More perniciously, it also revealed that the number of staff vacancies across the NHS hit new heights with 107,743 unfilled posts. It reported that the NHS was short of 41,722 nurses—11.8% of the nursing workforce—while nearly 1 in 10 doctor posts were vacant, and warned that the difficulties in recruiting and retaining staff were so serious the vacancies would worsen over the coming months.[4] The King's Fund verdict was: 'Widespread and growing nursing shortages now risk becoming a national emergency and are symptomatic of a long-term failure in workforce planning.'

Agency costs have rocketed, with the very same staff coming from the NHS accounting for approximately 80% of the nursing and medical shifts filled. While a little agency work is healthy, a total reliance on it filling vacancies and gaps is a serious and substantial shortcoming. Overworked, tired, and stressed staff cannot sustainably provide the care they would like to give. Resilience is weak, burnout is strong.

In 2016–2017 the House of Lords launched an investigation into the long-term sustainability of the NHS and adult social care and I, along with others, was asked to give evidence. Its report did not pull its punches, concluding: 'We are concerned by the absence of any comprehensive national long-term strategy to secure the appropriately skilled, well-trained and committed workforce that the health and care system will need over the next 10–15 years. In our view this represents the biggest internal threat to the sustainability of the NHS.' Getting to the heart of the problem, it added: 'We also heard repeatedly of the linkage between overburdensome regulation, unnecessary bureaucracy, a prolonged period of pay restraint, low levels of morale and retention problems.' It called for sweeping changes to the way education and training are organized, planned, and delivered.

Yet, it would be unfair to imply that politicians, health executives, and professional leaders have not noticed this problem and started to deal with it. In February 2018, the government accepted many of the points made in the report but reminded the House of Lords that extra funding had been committed and more staff had been employed. It stressed that its priority was to deliver improvements for patients while managing demand and achieving financial balance.

By March 2018, Health Education England (HEE), the body responsible for planning workforce numbers and paying for training, had closed consultations on its draft workforce strategy to 2027 and by July 2018, to celebrate the seventieth birthday of the NHS, the government announced extra funding for a new 10-year NHS plan which would see spending for NHS England rise by around £20 billion from £115 billion in 2018–2019 to £135 billion by 2023–2024; an increase of 3.4% in real terms.[5]

Seen from space

In 2012 the challenges facing the NHS were compounded by the government imposing structural reforms which then NHS England chief executive Sir David Nicholson famously described as being big enough to be seen from space. They established a complicated patchwork of central bodies controlling commissioning, hospitals, and regulation alongside a hugely fragmented system of GP-led clinical commissioning groups responsible for local services and a misguided reliance on market mechanisms to drive quality. They proved a major obstacle to closer working between primary, secondary, and social care. These reforms warrant serious reflection globally. Any system that forgets that 'there is no healthcare without a workforce' and overcomplicates its taxonomy and policies to obfuscate clear responsibilities and accountabilities will reap the consequences. While officials can point to some good actions, such as substantially increasing the number of medical and nursing school places (up by 25% for doctors) and injecting an extra £2.4 billion a year to help primary care, the policy and practice levers are both fragmented and disconnected and therefore much more difficult to execute.[6]

Since 2014 the guiding document for NHS management has been the Five Year Forward View, launched by NHS England. It set some refreshing aspirations for integrated care, strengthened primary care, more care in the community, greater patient empowerment, improved health promotion, and less reliance on hospital care. But patient demand continues to climb and, currently, the reality seems to be fewer general practitioners, more specialist hospital medical staff, fewer community nurses, inundated hospitals, and an emaciated and creaking social care system. There have been localized examples of integrated care with innovative clinical teams working in different ways to meet patient needs but delivering reform at speed and scale has been neither orchestrated nor leveraged.

The Long-Term Plan

Sensibly, in an attempt to provide a comprehensive and consolidated view of clinical strategy, services priorities, financing and workforce needs, the government took the decision to integrate all these issues into the new 10-year plan announced by the prime minister in June 2018 alongside the extra funding. It was a timely and much needed announcement and, while think tanks and others said the money fell short of the 4% real terms annual funding increase they believed was needed, it represented a vastly superior offer than all other spending priorities such as education, policing, defence, and social care.

And the offer needed to be big. The HEE consultation document was impressive in its factual detail, but two facts stood out. First, the retention rate of staff is falling. Like any leaky sieve, it doesn't matter how many training places you pour in if staff are going to leave through burnout and better career opportunities elsewhere. HEE stated 'the percentage of nurses leaving the NHS for reasons other than retirement increased from 7.1% in 2011/12 to 8.7% in 2016/17', adding that had the rate remained at 2012 levels there would be 16,000 more nurses working which would be almost half of the existing nurse vacancy rate. Second, and unprecedentedly, it asserted 'our ten year forward look shows that if no action is taken . . . the NHS will need to grow by 190,000 clinical posts by 2027 to meet demand'.[7] Roughly, that's an increase of over 15%, a feat that has never been achieved before.

But the Long Term Plan has given the NHS a new sense of hope and ambition. Recognising the difficulties over the previous decade, prime minister Theresa May unveiled the NHS England document in January 2019. She hailed the launch as a 'truly historic moment' and promised 'a new service model for the twenty-first century' which could save up to half a million lives by focussing on prevention and early detection of illness.

The plan set out six priority areas for progress over the coming decade, largely reflecting best practice innovations by other health systems noted elsewhere in this book but also building on smaller, local case studies initiated by the previous Five Year Forward View.

The most striking priority was the promise to grow investment in primary and community care services faster than the overall NHS budget, an extra £4.5 billion investment per year heralded as an 'NHS first'. This will enable more services to be provided by joined-up, integrated teams in primary, community and social care. Further, over the next five years, the plan promised patients the right to have digital

GP consultations while avoiding up to a third of hospital face-to-face outpatient attendances.

Second, the plan set out action the NHS will take to strengthen its contribution to prevention and reducing health inequalities by developing new evidence-based programmes in smoking, obesity, alcohol, diabetes and air pollution. It asks local health systems to draw up five- and ten-year plans to reduce health inequalities, echoing the excellent report by chief medical officer Professor Dame Sally Davies, Health 2040 - Better Health Within Reach, which argued powerfully that "we need to reposition health as one of the primary assets of our nation, contributing to both the economy and happiness".

Improvements to care quality and outcomes form the third priority, with new investments in maternity and neonatal services, children's, young people's and adult mental health, learning disability and autism, earlier detection in cancer and cardiovascular disease and stroke care, while recognising the importance of research and development to the national economy.

Priorities four, five and six concentrate on the strategies to make it all happen; workforce, technology and money. Sensitive to the criticism that the Five Year Forward View lacked a detailed implementation plan, the Long Term Plan identifies practical steps and states "we have taken account of the current financial pressures across the NHS, which are a first call on extra funds". It asks hospitals to be in financial balance by 2020/21 and requires all NHS organisations to be back in surplus by 2023/24, perhaps recognising the size of challenge that lies ahead post-Brexit, with reduced economic growth forecast.

Putting the workforce centre-stage

Acknowledging past mistakes and omissions, the Long Term Plan seeks to address workforce problems and emphasises that "the performance of any healthcare system ultimately depends on its people". It recognises the strains and pressures NHS staff currently face but, sadly, creates a rather inward-looking National Workforce Group which will only develop a workforce implementation plan 'later in 2019'. Separating the workforce strategy from the Long Term Plan has been driven by politics - the government will not set out the funding for healthcare staff education and training for several months. But this runs the serious risk that workforce planning focusses on staff supply and demand rather than giving equal weight to their productivity, motivation, culture and leadership. Workforce should not be separated from the plan but woven through every part of it.

The plan rightly calls for an increase in recruiting more doctors, nurses, midwives, allied health professionals, scientists and others and acknowledges that much more can be done for retention, working conditions and culture. The chief executive of NHS Providers, Chris Hopson, said: "This plan cannot be delivered whilst trusts have 100,000 workforce vacancies. We need urgent action to solve what trust leaders currently describe as their biggest problem. It's a major concern that we will have to wait longer to get the comprehensive plan that is needed."

But the absence of meaningful, tangible workforce actions which build productivity as well as total numbers to support the delivery of the Long Term Plan will remain its Achilles' Heel until resolved. The NHS will secure its biggest wins by motivating the mass of healthcare staff to develop a learning culture and the skills in quality improvement to drive up quality, safety and productivity for the long-term.

While political opposition parties and health think tanks have been quick to point out that total investment still falls behind historic NHS growth levels, that the plan avoids dealing with the crucial issue of social care, sets mightily challenging financial recovery plans for hospitals in distress and potentially pushes waiting times up further, it is the need for a radical, imaginative and long-term plan for the workforce that will make or break the laudable intentions of the new policy, designed to take the NHS to 2030. New policies don't provide better services unless staff feel wholeheartedly supported and empowered.

That said, the move to create Integrated Care Systems 'everywhere by April 2021' to enhance population health management across the NHS is a bold move and, in a wonderfully worded plea list of potential legislative changes noted at the back of the document to make the plan more effective, might just do away with the purchaser-provider separation created back in 1991 and ease away the more toxic elements of the Health and Social Care Act of 2012. That's politics for you but, right now, I doubt any pundits can accurately predict what will happen to the UK in the next year, let alone decade, given the turmoil of Brexit.

Chapter 15

AI, robotics and digital disruption—rise of the humans?

More than two decades ago IBM's Deep Blue computer demonstrated the coming power of machine learning by winning a chess match against world champion Garry Kasparov. Today, advances in robotics, artificial intelligence, and machine learning, in which machines mimic cognitive functions such as learning and problem solving, are ushering in a new age of automation as machines match or outperform humans in a range of work activities, including those requiring cognitive capabilities. A 2018 study published in *Nature* revealed that artificial intelligence has demonstrated an ability to interpret three-dimensional scans of the eye and make referral recommendations that reach or exceed that of experts for a range of sight-threatening retinal diseases, after training on only 14,884 scans.[1]

According to Boston Consulting Group, artificial intelligence—AI—is a broad term to describe machines that perform tasks characteristic of human intelligence. Machine learning is a subset of AI that uses data to train algorithms; in effect, enabling intelligence by allowing the algorithm to learn and adapt. Deep learning is a subset of machine learning, which mimics neural networks to allow learning from un-structured data as opposed to task-specific algorithms. Robotics is the technology behind robots programmed to perform a fixed set of tasks autonomously or semi-autonomously. AI-powered robots are a relatively small subset. Software bots, or just bots, are the software equivalent of robots, carrying out automated tasks. These can range from simple programmes right up to those chewing through vast amounts of information on a supercomputer.

While successive reports have vividly demonstrated automation will first come *en masse* to industries such as manufacturing, agriculture, and transport, healthcare is not immune from this irresistible disruption (see Fig. 15.1). Nor should it be. Automation can raise performance by reducing errors and improving quality and speed, and in some cases achieving outcomes beyond human capabilities. According to a Boston/MIT international survey, almost 60% of healthcare organizations ex-pect artificial intelligence to have a big effect within five years.[2]

Investing in automation at scale can enhance productivity. The McKinsey Global Institute suggests productivity could increase by nearly 50%, boosting the economy at a time of lacklustre productivity growth and helping offset the impact of a declining share of the population being of working age. They suggest that while only 5% of cur-rent workplace activities can be fully automated through existing technology, over half of all occupations could have about one-third of their work routines handled by machines.[3]

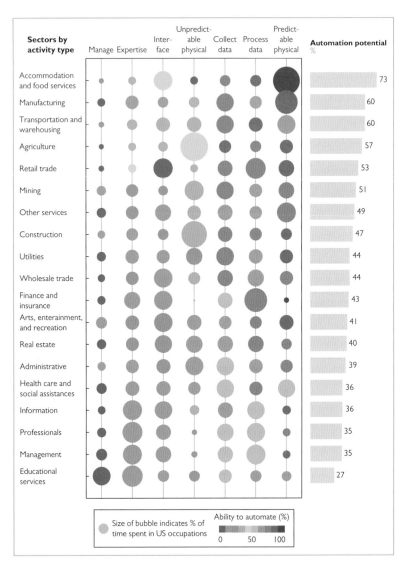

Fig. 15.1 Technical potential for automation across sectors varies depending on mix of activity types.

As McKinsey highlights, identifying precise productivity gains for healthcare from artificial intelligence is difficult, because it is one of the few industries where there is growing demand for manual as well as technological labour. It estimates that healthcare labour productivity across Western Europe and the United States fell by a compound average rate of about 1.2% between 2000 and 2016.

Much fear about robotics and artificial intelligence rightly concerns the displacement of human labour. While few commentators offer little more than platitudes about governments and businesses being socially responsible for ensuring a benign transition which mitigates the consequences, it is worth remembering that much of the healthcare workforce in the developed world is ageing and that it is all but certain that in the future we will have too few, not too many, workers. It is even questionable whether artificial intelligence will destroy more jobs than it creates. Gartner is just one organization predicting that there will be a net jobs gain in the next few years.

I have seen how robots are already providing aged care in Japan and Singapore, dispensing drugs in America and China, and cleaning and carrying supplies in hospitals in the Netherlands and Germany. Workforce typically accounts for 60–70% of a hospital's expenditure. I do not believe robots, artificial intelligence, or any combination of them will replace doctors, nurses, and care assistants anytime soon, but we often forget that administration absorbs a substantial proportion of hospital costs—typically around 25% in a US hospital, 16% in England, and 12% in Canada.[4] These include tasks such as coding and billing, which can be automated already.

New business models are desperately needed in areas which currently resemble nineteenth-century cottage industries, with staff being retrained as care assistants, care navigators, and case managers, thereby improving both care integration and patient empowerment, fundamental to improving productivity and quality.

Asking 'Will a robot or AI take my job?' is the wrong question. Generally, machines will take over tasks, not entire jobs. Radiologists are not in danger of being replaced by artificial intelligence, but machine learning will profoundly change their role by taking over much of the routine assessment of medical images, and do so with a lower error rate. So the challenge for healthcare systems is to redesign end-to-end processes to enable humans and machines to work together in a way that allows each to focus on the tasks at which they excel.[5] The end result may well be that staff move up the food chain, escaping routine but nonetheless error-prone work to focus on interpreting and responding to results produced by or with the aid of machines, building relationships with patients and managing their care.

While I do not believe automation will lead to substantial job losses among doctors and nurses, it will change the health workforce. As this new discipline develops, mid-range jobs such as technicians working in pathology laboratories will be most at risk, while at the upper end, healthcare will be in a fierce competition with other industries to attract and retain the technologists necessary to build, develop, and run systems.

Lifelong learning

To reflect this new world in which people and intelligent machines work side-by-side, commentators have begun to talk about a third form of intelligence. Alongside raw intellectual power (IQ) and emotional intelligence (EQ), they have added the robotic quotient—RQ, the extent to which we have the skills and attitudes to work symbiotically with machines. This idea rams home the point that, far from intelligent automation deskilling the clinical workforce, it adds another intellectual and cultural challenge to working in healthcare.

Intelligent automation will bring an even sharper intellectual edge to medical training and lifelong development. It will heighten the importance of learning to learn—acquiring the techniques and attitudes to enable the continual acquisition of new skills. Will the day come when the ability to work with machines will be part of the assessment of a doctor's fitness to practise?

The organizational challenge

The organizational challenge of all this is immense. Healthcare systems—not least the NHS—have often been accused of using technology to automate inefficiency rather than as an opportunity to design better ways of working. Simply trying to crowbar machine learning into existing organizational and care pathways will not work. It will lead to wasted investment, humans and machines duplicating activities, and above all, a failure to exploit machine learning to its full potential while liberating humans to doing what they do best—managing the care of their fellow humans. So jobs, teams, processes, and functions will need to be redesigned.

As the rate of change accelerates, healthcare systems will have to rethink and reorganize ever faster. Our performance to date in terms of rapidly, repeatedly rebuilding systems to exploit technology, is not promising.

When redesigning organizations and systems, leaders and teams will need to consider and reconcile an extraordinary range of factors. These include: what is possible with digital technology; which of the numerous technological possibilities will match the hype; which will work best in our organization; what skills and capabilities are needed to deliver that potential; which organizational models will work best in integrating human and machine intelligence; what is the right mix of permanent and gig economy workers; how should we approach workforce displacement and transition; how do we reform the education and training of our staff to be more responsive to the demands of the future workforce; and how can the organization redesign current roles to attract and retain talent with advanced technological skills?

This permanent revolution will create another workforce challenge—securing the skills and capacity to design and build organizational systems and care pathways which integrate machine learning and human activity, while constantly evolving and adapting as technology develops. The skills that will be needed include: design thinking—redesigning processes through the lens of patient experiences and outcomes; systems thinking—understanding the whole picture and the connections within it; creativity—being able to invent new organizational forms and services; data analysis—understanding the strengths and limitations of data, the difference between symptoms and causes and how to interpret evidence; and cognitive flexibility—switching between thinking about two different concepts, and thinking about multiple concepts simultaneously. All that is on top of the skills to design and implement the machine learning tools themselves.

There will be endless opportunities to get all this wrong. Organizations which maximize the chances of getting most of it right most of the time will focus on long-term goals rather than short-term costs, will have sufficient human, financial, and technical resources in place, will start small to gain experience and learn hard lessons, demonstrate some quick wins, and build momentum, will look at the end-to-end system rather than just a small part of the process, and will lead the project strategically rather than dump it on the IT department.

But as always it will be leadership, interpersonal skills, and emotional intelligence that will make or break this change. Automation will heighten the importance of the human touch. Providing staff with a compelling narrative about the benefits of intelligent automation for both patients and themselves will be crucial. If clinicians believe they are being undermined, undervalued, or replaced by machines, morale and performance will go into freefall.

The ever-changing workforce

The intelligent automation revolution makes health workforce planning ever more difficult. The old 'predict and provide' approach to estimating future workforce needs—never a great success—is wholly inadequate in the face of the advance of the robots. Healthcare organizations instead need to develop transition strategies to manage the disruption of their clinical workforce as automation repeatedly forces roles to be adapted and reinvented.

Agile workforce planning (see Fig. 15.2) will require a multifaceted view—the right balance between permanent staff and a more 'gig economy' approach, the right machine resources to run alongside the humans and an understanding of how this will change over time, and a more networked approach to career and skills development. [6] These are just some of the challenges.

Machine learning will inevitably be applied to the planning and management of the workforce itself. Greater understanding of patient flows and how to control them will lead to changes in the size, shape, and distribution of staffing through the days, weeks, and years. Monitoring the movement of porters around the hospital or nurses around the ward will open up new ways of organizing and working.

The risks of unleashing this technology on the workforce itself are immense. There is obviously the danger that staff will feel they are being monitored by a Big Brother. Managers and leaders will need to use information with care and sensitivity to avoid staff feeling they are having their privacy invaded and their contribution reduced to data which fails to reflect the relationship between clinicians and patients. This would destroy trust and engagement. Staff need to feel the benefits of intelligent automation, not feel they are being controlled by it, one of many causes of 'automation anxiety'.

Machine learning will also affect how staff are recruited and what recruiters are looking for when hiring clinicians and technologists alike. In the recruitment process,

From: Strategic workforce planning	To: Agile workforce shaping
Supply and demand analysis looking and 'gap closing' over a three- to five-year time horizon	Continuous analysis of workforce impact and required skills as intelligent automation is deployed
Analysis based on existing job families	Analysis based on job families and new required capabilities based on 'to-be' tasks and critical skills for end-to-end processes
Owned and conducted by HR, which consults with the business	Owned and conducted by the business units and end-to-end process owners, facilitated by HR
Employed workers	Human workers both employed and not employed as well as bots owned and not owned
Traditional pyramidal top-down work structures with critical roles driven by hierarchy	Team-based and an end-to-end process view of work organization with critical roles driven by skill scarcity and value-add to the business
Bias for 'an answer' with sensitivity analysis on either side based on existing organization mindset	Bias for scenarios with probabilities attached, based on horizon scanning and "outside-in" mindset
Current workforce model (shape and structure of the workforce in terms of spans, layers, rates of attrition and promotion, etc.) provides the dominant mental model for the planning effort	Ongoing reexamination of the workforce model using a framework such as the 5Cs to ensure a more multidisciplinary approach to forecasting and the possibilities for the organization

Fig. 15.2 Strategic workforce planning to agile workforce shaping.

artificial intelligence will increasingly play a role in identifying suitable candidates with online testing of their abilities. As the importance of these skills grows, health employers will need to collaborate with other organizations to find and keep the right talent. In terms of the skills needed, as Kevin Green, CEO of What's Next Consultancy points out, the emphasis will shift from knowledge and experience to demonstrating an ability to solve problems, think creatively, and adapt to new environments.[7]

Attracting tech talent

The risk for healthcare is that automation creates a workforce shortage in technology alongside all the difficulties in recruiting clinical staff. According to a McKinsey Global Institute study of five industries across Western Europe and the United States, healthcare and retail will experience the biggest shift towards technological skills, ahead of manufacturing, banking and insurance, and energy and mining. Growth will be driven by ever-growing connectivity to deliver patient co-management, real-time analytics, and automation. McKinsey predicts major growth in demand for advanced IT skills, basic digital skills, entrepreneurship, and adaptability, while demand for skills such as inspecting and monitoring patients' vital signs and medical equipment will stagnate as machines take over routine tasks. So healthcare will face a big scramble for tech talent.

Part of the problem will no doubt be paying enough to attract that talent, but the critical factor will be the working environment. Healthcare organizations have to become far more attractive. The social value of working in healthcare and the human skills they will learn may well help recruit people, but they will not be enough to keep them. One of the biggest challenges will be to provide technologists with a learning environment, where they are able to acquire new skills and have hands-on experience of the latest technological developments. If they feel they are falling behind their peers by being forced to work on outdated systems, they will leave. Therefore retention will be key.

IT recruitment experts increasingly talk about the importance of the brand image and values around technology when it comes to people choosing potential employers; it is easy to imagine that within a few years world-leading healthcare institutions will be defined as much by the technologists they attract as the doctors. They will need to be recognized as far more than a backroom function. A supportive, well-resourced working environment needs to be part of the deal.

The difficulties of machine learning in the real world

It is important to recognize the risks when incorporating machine learning into clinical decision-making. Many of the systems on which healthcare will depend will be clinical decision support systems. These hold out the prospect of being able to shorten greatly the time it takes for research to influence clinical practice by sifting through the hundreds of thousands of research papers published each year to identify relevant data, and adapting their assessments of illnesses and treatments over time as they learn from changes in population and disease trends.

But researchers have identified significant difficulties in moving these amazing systems from clinical trials to everyday use in hospitals and clinics.[8] While they can work well in simulations, the only test that really matters is patient outcomes. When these systems are being assessed for clinical use, this needs to be done with the same rigour as other medical devices such as scanners. Isaac Asimov's first law for robots is 'do no harm'. Silicon Valley physician and tech entrepreneur Jordan Shlain points out that Facebook founder Mark Zuckerberg's approach of 'move fast and break things' won't work in healthcare. The mantra needs to be 'move slow and don't kill people'.[9]

The practical difficulties of implementing the systems is immense. In 2016 IBM's Watson system was credited with diagnosing in minutes a leukaemia patient whose condition had been baffling doctors for months, after cross-referencing her information with 20 million oncology records.[10] Hospitals are now beginning to introduce this sort of technology, but it can go wrong. The University of Texas MD Anderson Cancer Center consumed $62 million over five years struggling to integrate AI into its clinical work.[11] Many healthcare systems—including the NHS—are still trying to implement comprehensive electronic healthcare records. Implementing intelligent automation is many times harder, and a world away from the plug and play systems we take for granted as consumers.

A key obstacle to assessing the reliability of intelligent automation is the 'black box problem', in that the networks in their algorithms are so complex that the user may be unable to understand how the machine came to a decision.[12] The risk is that a clinician may be more inclined to support a wrong decision because it has come from a machine, rather than a more obviously fallible colleague. Automation does not negate the importance of clinical judgement. It also presents a monumental problem for regulators in assessing the safety of automated systems, not least because manufacturers are reticent to reveal their intellectual secrets.

Climbing in the foothills

Techemergence.com has looked at how five of the top hospitals in the United States are trying to develop machine learning. So far, the applications focus on predictive analytics—assessing patients to anticipate and prevent emergencies—as well as predictive health trackers to monitor patients' health status in real time and chatbots to provide automated responses to physicians' enquiries.[13]

One example cited—very much in its development phase—is the Mayo Clinic's Center for Individualized Medicine collaboration with a health tech start-up called Tempus. They are carrying out molecular sequencing and analysis for around 1,000 patients for several cancer types including lung cancer and melanoma, with the aim of delivering more customized immunotherapy treatments.[14] Several universities are part of the same consortium, highlighting the collaborative nature of advances in machine learning.

At the Cleveland Clinic, a collaboration with Microsoft—using the technology behind Cortana, Microsoft's AI digital assistant—aims to identify patients in intensive care (ICU) at high risk of cardiac arrest.[15] Massachusetts General Hospital is training a supercomputer using billions of medical images to identify applications in radiology and pathology.[16] So even the world's leading hospitals are still scrambling around in the foothills of machine learning—but with huge ambitions.

Displacing administrative staff—to do what?

Industries such as the utilities and financial services have already transformed their back and middle office functions by centralizing facilities and standardizing and optimizing processes to reduce errors and waste. In recent years they have been investing heavily in robotic process automation (RPA) using software robots to automate routine functions, which is already moving from standardized, structured processes into intelligent automation using unstructured information. According the Professor Leslie Willcocks and others at the London School of Economics, robotic automation particularly lends itself to 'swivel chair' functions such as on-boarding a new employee, where traditionally a member of staff has interacted with numerous computer systems to perform functions such as setting up an email account and issuing a security pass.[17] Such systems can automate numerous tasks (including bureaucratic ones with which clinicians are currently lumbered), and are technically reasonably straightforward to set up.

Private healthcare organizations may well use this technological power simply to cut costs, but for public health systems it provides the opportunity to move staff from being an administrative cost to adding value to patient experiences and outcomes. As we have seen in the chapter on patients and carers as partners, empowering patients to drive change in value in the healthcare system requires new roles to support patients in managing their conditions and in making decisions about their care. Healthcare organizations should be retraining administrative staff—not making them redundant—and bringing them in to patient facing roles. The staff should be seen as having great potential as agents of system change, not just simply a cost to be stripped out. By working in healthcare they have already absorbed the values of their organizations and contribute to the patient experience and outcomes. This is a great example of how healthcare should be supporting lifelong training and learning.

Blockchain

Blockchain is open source software where digital units (of money or data) are organized into a series of chronologically grouped transactions, or blocks, which are digitally signed. The technology behind blockchain involves cryptography, coding, and networking, managed by sophisticated mathematical algorithms. The power of blockchain is that it allows organizations to provide access to secured content selectively in a trusted and controlled mechanism. At the same time, they can prevent copying or destruction of data and record 'one version of the truth'—such as an electronic patient record—that can be cryptographically proven to be correct. Blockchain is not fast, but it provides what John Halamka, chief information officer of Beth Israel Deaconess Medical Center in Boston, calls 'a tamperproof public ledger'.[18]

Halamka told Forbes that among the benefits for healthcare, a blockchain medical record provides absolute proof and confidence that it cannot be changed once it is generated and signed—a principle that can also be applied to clinical trials. It is also ideally suited to managing consent for sharing medical information—anyone seeking to exchange medical data about a patient would check the blockchain for permission to do so. In a world of increasing sensitivity about privacy and sharing, blockchain could be revolutionary in allowing patients to control their data while ensuring everyone who needs access can get it.

The power of blockchain extends to intelligent medical devices, wearables, bio sensors, and other connected devices which create continuous sensitive data streams. Distributed ledger technologies like blockchain could be the basis of security mechanisms that include time-stamped audit trails to verify and validate the authenticity of data streams. Healthcare has been slow to the blockchain party but its potential is vast.

Don't get left behind

One of the biggest risks I see with AI is that it could easily lead to an ever-widening gap between the most advanced healthcare institutions and systems and the rest.

The disparity may become most apparent within a particular system, with many institutions struggling to get to grips with the idea and attract the talent to deliver it while the best resourced, most ambitious, and most respected hospitals disappear into the distance as they build ground-breaking alliances with big tech firms and exciting start-ups.

No hospital can do this alone. They need to work together across regions, countries, and continents to share ideas, solutions, and talent. They also need to remember what they bring to their relationship with the technology companies. The technologists cannot achieve anything without the data and clinical know-how of the healthcare providers, so health institutions need to make sure they get their fair share of any commercial success. Meanwhile the preparations for AI need to begin now, starting with the rewriting of every clinical syllabus and a much better appreciation and analysis of the tasks people actually do—work as done, not imagined.

Chapter 16

Japan—centenarians and robots

British prime minister of the Victorian era, Benjamin Disraeli, once said: 'Like all great travellers, I have seen more than I remember and remember more than I have seen.' Flying from one country to another I know I can sometimes misremember places and events—but not in Japan. It is a sensory feast; its culture, history, people, and societal structure leave an indelible mark in the memory.

Japan has proud traditions but is also highly evolved technologically, advancing robotics to new levels, particularly in the care of older people in a country with an extraordinary long lifespan. I have seen centenarians cuddle robotic seals and robots giving exercise classes. I love the idea that some of the earliest and most enthusiastic adopters of robotics may well be among the oldest people on the planet.

But Japan's fascination with robotics is not just driven by its extraordinary prowess in electronics—it has a workforce crisis affecting the entire economy. The 'three arrows' of prime minister Shinzo Abe's economic strategy (so-called Abenomics—monetary easing, fiscal stimulus, and structural reforms) have stimulated growth, but coupled with a shrinking working age population that means Japan is now at pretty much full employment. So increasing the supply of health workers from domestic stock will be a challenge. It may not even be desirable. Health is hardly the most productive part of the economy, and with the country worrying about growth, Japan's government will be thinking carefully about how to allocate its scarce workforce between sectors.

The obvious answer is immigration, but ministers have been unsure: 'Before accepting immigrants or refugees we need to have more activities by women, elderly people and we must raise our birth rate,' Abe has said.

Nonetheless, in 2018 the government announced there would be half a million visas for people willing to work in nursing, construction, agriculture, hotels, and shipbuilding. A step change? Unlikely. Dr Yasuhiro Suzuki, vice minister for health and chief medical and global health officer, told me the government sees Japan's steep growth in health demand as more of a hump. In 2025, he said, the last of the baby boomers will turn 75 and that hump will peak. By then it is hoped that policies to reduce demand, increase supply, and boost productivity will have started to build steam. The use of migrant labour is more of a temporary measure while those polices bed in.

The scale of the workforce problem

Japan's health workforce problem is big. Fortunately, it is so big they saw it coming and have not sat idly by. Japan's population is 127 million. In 40 years' time, it is

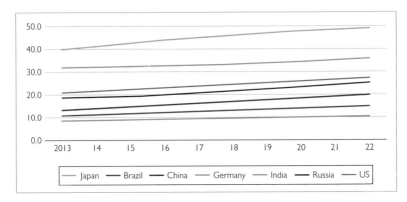

Fig. 16.1 Old-age dependency ratio, international comparison.
Reproduced with permission from The Economist Intelligence Uni. (2018) Industry Report Healthcare Japan. 1st Quarter 2018. © 2018 The Economist Intelligence Unit Limited.

expected to have fallen by a third. That might not have been a big problem for health if it were not for the shifting balance between generations. The over-65s will grow from 26% of the population to nearly 40%.[1] Meanwhile the working age population will shrink at about 1% a year.[2] Supporting Japan's elderly population is placing a growing financial and physical strain on its younger generations (see Fig. 16.1)—where there were just nine over-65s per 100 working age people in 1960, by 2017 there were 45.[3]

The shrinking population is a contracting force on the economy and puts pressure on a dwindling cohort of workers to work harder, even just to stand still. This is exactly what has been happening. While gross domestic product (GDP) as a whole stutters, GDP per working age person is second only to Germany.[4] Japanese workers cannot go on like this forever. Karoshi, the phenomenon of death by overwork, is a growing problem.

Increasing supply—women, pensioners, and robots

Japan has few doctors compared with other Organisation for Economic Co-operation and Development (OECD) countries and slightly more nurses. The OECD average per 1,000 population is around 3.2 doctors and 9.2 nurses; Japan has 2.4 doctors and 11.3 nurses.[5,6] Vacancy rates make clear that there are not enough of either, but the most desperate need is for care workers.

There were about 1.7 million care workers in 2013. This was a huge improvement—triple the 550,000 they had back in 2000.[7] The growth followed the introduction of long-term care insurance in 2000 and the subsequent expansion in nursing home capacity. There is pressure to keep the care workforce growing but it is difficult. The Japanese government estimates it will need 50% more again by 2025. On the current trajectory, it thinks it will achieve about half that, leaving them about 380,000 short. That is probably optimistic. Care facilities are full and there are long waiting lists. There is even a term for the thousands of elderly people who die alone in their homes every year—kodokushi—'silent death'.

Government plans to address this issue revolve around bringing those currently outside the workforce back in, especially women and older workers. Policies to raise female participation rates have already borne fruit. Until recently, female participation tended to have two peaks—early and later in life—and dip in the middle when many took time off work to have children. Recent data suggests that 'm-shaped curve' may now be flattening. Participation rates for women aged 30–34 rose to 75% in 2017—up from about 50% 30 years ago—and the participation rate for all working age women (15–64) rose to a record 69% in 2017. That year the government announced plans to build on the progress by creating enough children's day care centres to allow 80% of women aged 25–44 to work by 2020.

In an effort to extend people's working lives, the government plans to increase the retirement age to 65 in 2025, although they almost need not bother. The actual age men retire is closer to 70. Dr Shigeaki Hinohara—until recently the world's oldest practising clinician—was still doing daily rounds of his patients at 105 years old. In a recent report, McKinsey suggests that older workers might be well suited to some of the less intensive nursing care work, and according to a 2013 government survey, 11% of seniors who wanted to carry on working said they would be willing to do this kind of job. McKinsey calculates that if 10% of unemployed seniors in the 65–74 age range worked several days a week as nursing care staff, Japan could have 700,000 additional caregivers by 2025.[8]

However, despite success in recruiting more women and elders into the wider workforce, recruiting and retaining them in caring positions has proved tougher. Care workers are in high demand and short supply, yet homes say they are only able to offer wages significantly below the all-industry average, and it can be hard work. As a result, turnover is high, training facilities struggle to fill places, and in 2017 there were 3.5 carer positions for every jobseeker.[9] Since 2015 the government has tried to help care wages catch up, but with limited success.

Could robotics be the answer? Japanese industry is investing heavily in them (see Fig. 16.2). In 2012, soon after coming to office, Abe set aside Y2.39bn (around US$21m) to subsidize the development of nursing care robots.[10] Since then the Ministry for Economy, Trade, and Industry has invested in everything from self-driving toilets to talking seals. Japan's older people seem receptive so maybe this is the future, but robots will not solve the immediate crisis.

Japan needs migrant workers now—hence the recent visa announcement. Even that is only likely to be a short-term solution. A report last year from Merrill Lynch warns that a policy of importing labour, although helpful, 'will eventually hit a wall', so companies need to find more innovative business models.[11]

Increasing productivity

Successive governments have been keen to increase workforce productivity, so much so that, despite five prime ministers in five years, health and social welfare

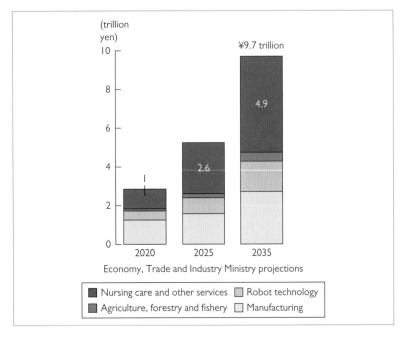

Fig. 16.2 Fastest-growing markets for robots by industry.

reforms between 2008 and 2012 were swept through on a wave of cross-party support, culminating in 2013 with the Social Security Reform Programme Act.

Like other countries, Japan is seeking to develop a more primary care-led, integrated health and social care service, through devolving power, budgets, and planning to regions. It is finding it tough going.

Historically, Japan has had an undifferentiated health service. At last count it had 8,442 hospitals and 101,529 clinics.[12] It only recently made a distinction between acute-specialty and long-term care beds, and the distinction between specialty and primary care doctors is even more vague. Early in their career most doctors choose a hospital specialty, later moving out to smaller hospitals and clinics where they provide both specialty and primary care services. General practice only became a specialty in its own right in 2017, so most practitioners do this kind of work alongside their other specialty without ever undergoing additional primary care training.

There are huge shortages in some hospital specialties, such as emergency medicine. This is partly because of staff moving to clinics but also because of the mix of primary and secondary work that specialists end up doing. Until recently there has been no centralized planning to ensure optimal allocation of doctors between professions.

There is no obligation for patients to seek advice from a primary care practitioner before requesting a specialty appointment, as the Fee For Service structure will reimburse both, so there are no official referral guidelines between primary and secondary care, no clear licensing credentials to distinguish primary care doctors, no integrated information systems, and no primary care quality indicators.[13]

Despite this, as a starting point for primary care-led, integrated care systems, the existing infrastructure is not bad. There are plenty of clinics, many well equipped for X-rays, electrocardiography and blood and urine tests, and the clinics with inpatient beds function as small community hospitals. But a lot of work will be required to get where they want to be.

The Social Security Reform Programme has done a great job mapping out that process, but the practicalities are proving difficult. Local governments have been asked to draw up their 'regional healthcare vision' of what integrated care services might look like in five years' time. Healthcare organizations have been asked to form local networks to optimize capacity and resource allocation. Regulations governing service quality have been tightened and hospitals must now present regular performance reports to local prefectures.

However, the process is butting up against the same issues that plague integrated care systems elsewhere. How do you get all these people around a table to thrash out competing interests and reach agreement? As ever, legislation is just the start—people need to make it happen.

Reducing demand—what needs to change?

There is plenty Japan can do to reduce demand for its health services. The average hospital stay at 16 days is three times the OECD average, and the average number of physician visits a year is also nearly twice the OECD average at 12.8.[14,15] Japan has almost three times more hospital beds per 1,000 population than most other developed nations.[16]

Facilitating this oversupply has been weak governance of medical practice. Their medical colleges are legion, guidelines frequently contradict each other, and doctors retain a lot of autonomy in how they diagnose and treat. Until recently they could pretty much prescribe what they wanted—from cold remedies to complementary medicine—and still expect reimbursement. It is astonishing that the country which brought us Toyota's lean method has done so little to standardize medicine.

Conclusion

In the government report *Japan Vision: Health Care 2035* I was surprised to see a focus on global health, particularly the development of universal health coverage.

It is one of only three core objectives for their health system. When I asked vice minister for health and chief medical officer Dr Suzuki about this, he told me that as a country whose military is focussed on self-defence, being good global neighbours has become key to their security strategy. What an innovative use of soft power, and what a contrast with the government's more insular immigration policy. It seems to me Japan's workforce policies mirror the fascinating contradictions I see elsewhere in Japanese society—traditional and innovative, isolationist and outward looking, simple and complex.

Japan's determination to exploit robotics as part of the solution to its workforce crisis exemplifies ideas which the rest of the world should embrace. It shows how imagination and drive can find solutions to even the most overwhelming problems, but it also demonstrates how public investment in healthcare creates both health and wealth. Japan has spotted that care of older people is a vast potential market for its technologically advanced products, and is already trialling these in 5,000 care homes. Robotics will swiftly make a big difference to the quality of life of many Japanese, while providing its industry with yet another outstanding export.

Chapter 17

The United States of America—disunited states

The United States never ceases to amaze me. Every time you think you know it, it changes. Not only because each of its 50 states has a distinctive culture and history but because its politics, economy, and defence systems shape the world order. I don't think I have spent time in a more openly polarized society, and this is reflected in its health systems. It can deliver the finest healthcare to some and yet leave millions without insurance. It is the only Organisation for Economic Co-operation and Development (OECD) country without universal health coverage but leads the world in research. Walter Cronkite, the famous TV anchor, once said 'America's healthcare system is neither healthy, caring, nor a system',[1] but it's difficult to generalize because of the uneven, mosaic-like distribution of staff and services that constitute it.

Geographical imbalances

Surprisingly the United States has a slightly low density of physicians with 2.6 per 1,000 population compared with the OECD average of 3.0,[2] but this aggregate figure hides shortfalls and surpluses across the country spanning specialties, regions, and income brackets. For example, there are huge variations in physician density. Despite nearly a fifth of US residents living in rural areas less than a tenth of primary care physicians work there, and the situation is worse for specialists. The National Rural Health Association reports that while there are 263 specialists per 100,000 residents in urban areas, there are just 30 in rural ones.[3]

The reasons for the gap are common to most large countries—lack of income potential in rural areas, the complex nature of the job, lack of employment opportunities for spouses, and a lack of good schools. The United States has been a test bed of policies to try to address them but efforts to date have been piecemeal and uncoordinated. The government body responsible for addressing the issue is the Department of Health and Human Services, which was recently criticised by the Government Accountability Office for devolving power to its various agencies and then failing to maintain comprehensive oversight of the 72 programmes carried out in its name.

To be fair, regional variation is hard to crack in the United States. Upstream measures to correct imbalances such as improved recruitment and training in underserved areas require the coordination and cooperation of states—difficult in a federated country—and downstream measures face challenges too. Inherent barriers to labour mobility makes re-licensing of existing staff across state borders difficult. Nursing scope of practice legislation is unique in each state and there can be multiple professional bodies for just one profession, with not all states recognizing all professional bodies.

Telehealth and remote monitoring technologies make the best use of existing staff no matter where they are, but it is still not the easy option. Differences in state law can make consulting across state borders troublesome, though federal government is working hard to harmonize this legislation. It would be a coup if it works, because in the words of cardiologist and digital medicine expert Dr Eric Topol, 'there's never going to be enough paediatric gastroenterologists in North Dakota'.[4]

Specialty imbalances

According to OECD data the United States has a good supply of specialists, ranking 13th out of 29 countries for specialist physician density. But it ranks poorly for general practitioners, coming 30th out of 31.[5] The difference between generalists and specialists is so large that only Greece has a more disparate ratio. Just 12% of medics are family doctors in the United States compared with 88% practising specialties.

If you look at physician incomes, it is not hard to see why some specialties are more popular than others. According to Medscape's 2018 Physician Compensation Report, orthopaedic surgeons earned an average $497k a year, compared with $212k a year for paediatricians.[6] Remuneration is key to determining specialty choice because of the vast debt doctors amass in training. The Association of American Medical Colleges reports the median education debt of a new medical school graduate is $190,000, while 14% of medical graduates start residency training owing more than $300,000. Most OECD countries subsidize medical training more.

There also tends to be more regulation of postgraduate training in other countries. In the United Kingdom, for example, training places for specialties are limited and, as far as possible, evenly distributed across the country. In the United States, by contrast, weak governance of the Graduate Medical Education process means doctors can easily 'follow the money' into lucrative specialties. The effect is a workforce that reflects the needs of the profession better than that of the population and when the profession is still largely reimbursed through fee-for-service, it is not hard to see why cost inflation is rampant.

A report on medical education by the Institute of Medicine in 2014 described how outdated funding mechanisms perpetuated outdated workforce dynamics and hindered progress to new models of care. The institute report received support from a number of high-profile organizations including the Commonwealth Fund, Aetna Foundation, and Kaiser Permanente Institute for Health Policy, all worried about the appropriateness of the future physician workforce. It also received public endorsement from the Government Accountability Office, who used the findings to criticise the health department again for its oversight of medical education.

One of the report's recommendations was for better governance of what is a large sum of public money—$16.3 billion was spent on graduate medical education in 2015—but currently governments do little to leverage that payment to get the workforce they need. Such changes would require legislation and so far there has been little appetite for it.

In the absence of a centrally coordinated strategy, some organizations have taken matters into their own hands. Kaiser Permanente, a not-for-profit accountable care organization (ACO), has recently set up its own medical school, building the workforce it needs for its primary care-led and population health-based models. New York University School of Medicine recently announced it is offering all students fully funded scholarships regardless of merit or need, so they are able to 'choose a specialty based on their talent and inclinations to better serve the communities who need it most'.

The examples highlight the best of American innovation and philanthropy but are the exception, not the norm—most organizations lack the size, status, and resource to behave so radically.

The future

There is widespread disagreement in the United States about whether there will be a physician shortage. The Association of American Medical Colleges thinks there will. In 2015, it projected a shortfall of 45,400 primary care physicians by 2020.[7] That same year however, the Health Resources and Services Administration predicted a shortfall of 6,400,[8] while think tank the Cecil G. Sheps Center for Health Services Research thought that overall supply would be adequate.[9]

The forecasts vary so much because of different assumptions about future models of care. The optimists think that greater adoption of technology, a wider skill mix, and redesigned pathways of care mean there will be enough. The pessimists think it unlikely. Who you believe depends on the extent to which you think the United States will be able to adopt new models of care. The answer is probably somewhere between those rose-tinted and sceptical extremes. The last big attempt to encourage new models of care was the Affordable Care Act (ACA) in 2010 but uptake has been only partial. As of June 2018, 15 out of 50 states opted out of the legislation and only 26 of the remaining states and Washington DC have gone on to expand Medicaid coverage.[10]

Accompanying workforce transformation has also been patchy. While some states fully exploited the ACA's opportunities, others have been half-hearted. In 2010, for instance, Michigan bid for $9.8 million of ACA workforce transformation funding to spend on nurse education. Some $1.4 million went to Michigan State University to expand their advanced nurse practitioner programme, and Spectrum Health received $3.5 million to expand their primary care residency programme.[11] But while Michigan has spent transformation capital on training programmes, others have spent it on new hires with no plans for how to fund those new hires when the one-off funding runs out.

An imminent nursing crisis also threatens new models of care (see Fig. 17.1). Although the current density of nurses in the United States is on a par with other OECD countries at 11.6 per 1,000 population, it is estimated nearly a third of nurses will reach retirement age in the next 10–15 years.[12]

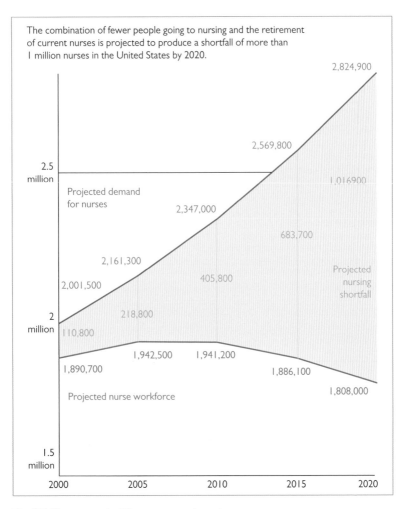

Fig. 17.1 There are too few US nurses to meet demand.

Reproduced with permission from Vy, P. States Work to Avert Nurse Shortage. Stateline. September 22, 2008. Copyright ©2008 The Pew Charitable Trusts. Available at http://www.pewtrusts.org/en/research-and-analysis/blogs/stateline/2008/09/22/states-work-to-avert-nurse-shortage

Though enrolments are up, it is unlikely to be sufficient. The American Association of Colleges of Nursing predicts a million new nurses will be needed by 2020. Expansion in training numbers has been limited by a lack of faculty staff to provide teaching.[13] In the short term, employers are responding to the nursing crisis by trying to buy their way out of trouble with offers of big bonuses, free housing, and free tuition for potential recruits.

Numbers are not enough

It seems likely the United States will require substantially more doctors and nurses in future than are currently due to materialize. In the past they have tended to import them—the number of residency slots vastly outweighs the number of graduating MDs every year and foreign-trained doctors and nurses more commonly work in underserved areas than their domestically trained counterparts. How palatable (or possible) that will be under the Trump administration is open to debate, however.

Simply boosting graduate numbers will not help either unless there are measures in place to ensure a more even spread. President Reagan tried that in the 1980s, but despite increasing per capita physician supply by 45% for primary care doctors, 188% for medical specialists, and 21% for surgical specialists in 20 years, it made almost no difference to those that needed it most. The new doctors flocked to the same places as the old ones—rich, urban areas with plenty of scope for private practice, with four out of five new physicians settling in regions where supply was already high.[14] Numbers are not enough. Skill mix and distribution are just as important if they are to turn health workers into health outcomes.

Cost and affordability

Even if the United States managed to achieve such a workforce, however, cost and ability to pay limits access to clinicians in the United States. Around twice as many Americans report having missed an appointment due to cost and around 10% of the population is uninsured, with many more underinsured.[15] A recent article in the *Journal of the American Medical Association (JAMA)* comparing the United States with other high-income countries found it had the most inequitable access to physicians when adjusted for need.[16]

Escalating health costs threaten to erode access to clinicians further (see Fig. 17.2). With spending on health accounting for 17.9% of American gross domestic product (GDP),[17] healthcare costs are now the major driver of national debt and deficits. Because, despite being thought of as the epitome of the private health insurance model, US federal subsidies of insured persons totalled $685bn in 2018 and in just 10 years' time that number is expected to almost double to $1.2 trillion. By that point, health spending will be the largest component of a federal debt amounting to 100% of GDP. By 2048, the Congressional Budget Office thinks it could be 152%.[18]

Successive governments have tried to control health expenditure. Obamacare, as well as expanding health insurance cover, also legislated to contain costs. Medicare will receive $716 billion less over the first 10 years of the ACA as a result of cuts to nursing services, a switch from fee-for-service to value-based payments and caps on insurance plan cost increases.[19] Medicaid has been subject to similar payment reform.

The ACA reforms have focused mainly on volume control, but unit cost of services is also important and has been less comprehensively addressed. A recent *JAMA* article looked at common procedures in the United States such as

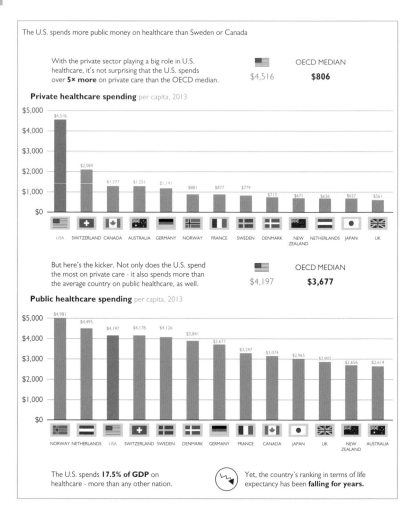

Fig. 17.2 Sticker shock.

Reproduced with permission from Desjardins, J. The U.S. Spends More Public Money on Healthcare Than Sweden or Canada. Visual Capitalist. March 31, 2017. Copyright © 2017 Visual Capitalist. Available at http://www.visualcapitalist.com/u-s-spends-

hip replacements and angioplasties, and found similar use rates per head of the population to comparable high-income countries.[20] This implies that the high costs are not the result of doing more, just costing more, from pharmaceuticals and MRI scans to consulting. The costs reflect more than just the products and procedures on an itemized hospital bill, however. They also reflect the bloated and bureaucratic system that lies beneath it.

Breaking the mould

Blitzing bloated bureaucratic systems is not something governments are usually known for, but a wave of innovative disruption bubbling up in the American healthcare system may have more success. Amazon, for example, is threatening the traditional pharmacy model by offering to deliver pharmaceuticals by drone, with the intention of reducing pharmaceutical costs and potentially freeing up pharmacists to do more face-to-face work.[21]

The proposed merger of CVS, America's biggest retail pharmacy, with Aetna, one of the biggest US health insurers, has been seen as a direct response to this development. By vertically integrating payer and provider, CVS-Aetna hope to shed layers of bureaucracy and cost and develop a strong retail primary care model with greater roles for non-physician staff. Currently CVS operates around 1,000 MinuteClinics across its 9,700 stores, offering basic low-cost health services to its customers. In partnership with Aetna however, it wants to expand into everything from diagnostics to dialysis (see Fig. 17.3).

The difference is data. With Aetna on board, CVS has better access to patients' medical files, enabling them to provide more complex, integrated care. In return Aetna benefits from lower cost care for its patients—fewer emergency room visits, better prevention of ill health, and better care coordination. With health cost inflation sitting around 6–7% in the United States, these are large stakes. The hope is that those cost savings will be passed on to consumers through lower premiums.

Aetna would also benefit because of CVS's role as a pharmacy-benefit manager (PBM). PBMs are a kind of middleman negotiating cost through bulk-buying pharmaceuticals on behalf of insurers. To give an idea of the potential for this kind of merger, consider what happened when UnitedHealth acquired a PBM in 2015. The new in-house PBM, named OptumRx, was able to take advantage of access to both medical files and pharmacy records, using data analytics and artificial intelligence (AI) to track medications use and effectiveness (and thereby making headway into personalized medicine). An article in *The Economist* expressed hope that this deal, if successful, could become a template for a new, lower cost ecosystem of quality healthcare.[22] I hope so.

Finally, the forthcoming not-for-profit set up between J.P. Morgan, Amazon, and Berkshire Hathaway will be one to watch. The three companies are planning to pilot a new health system tackling both insurance and provider issues. In addition, they have hired a leader with the right values—surgeon and public health expert Atul Gawande. The companies have said they will focus on their own employees and dependants for the time-being—thought to total a million people that roughly mirror wider US demographics—and will seek to tackle fraud, administration, chronic care, and end-of-life services to improve outcomes, harness the power of technology, and reduce costs. They are taking on many vested interests; as

Components of care delivery model

	Access to care	Patient engagement	Alignment across providers	Post-discharge
Pain points in current model	Inconvenient and inaccessible healthcare delivery system	Insufficient time to fully manage patient population	Lack of coordination to address gaps in care/unaligned inventives	Lack of support after a medical event
Ways CVS Health + Aetna can improve	Convenient locations and 'last mile' presence In-home and local community-based care	New forms of patient interactions to supplement physician office visits Enhanced consumer experience	Value-based provider relationships Combined pharmacy and medical data—single source for patient records	Transitions of care, along with care coaches/pharmacists and other programs

Fig. 17.3 CVS Health + Aetna can help better manage medical costs for chronic patients.
Reproduced with permission from Aetna and CVS Health. (2017) CVS Health + Aetna: Revolutionizing the Consumer Health Care Experience. Copyright © 2017 Aetna, Inc. Available at https://seekingalpha.com/article/4131025-cvs-and-aetna-risks-worth-rewards

Warren Buffet said, 'the resistance will be unbelievable and if we fail, at least we have tried'.

Conclusion

The United States truly is a unique and amazing place. President Franklin D. Roosevelt once said: 'Remember, remember always that all of us, and you and I especially, are descended from immigrants and revolutionists,' while Lyndon B. Johnson observed at the signing of the Immigration Bill in 1965: 'Our beautiful America was built by a nation of strangers . . . The land flourished because it was fed from so many sources— because it was nourished by so many cultures and traditions and peoples.'

America celebrates success, fails fast, learns quickly, and rarely gives up. It has been the incubator of many health and life science innovations which have helped its citizens and patients around the world. Yet, its fee-for-service payment model is now anachronistic to the model of care it needs. There is experimentation in both the public and private sectors and it may be that America's employers prove to be the most successful disruptors over the next decade because they are no longer prepared to see health cost inflation outstrip national economic growth. But make no mistake—historically, America has always been able to buy its way out of recruitment difficulties, and could do so again.

Chapter 18

Universal healthcare in our lifetime? All teach, all learn

The global movement around universal health coverage (UHC) has gathered momentum at blistering speed. Within a few years it has transformed the focus of healthcare in low- and middle-income countries from a few diseases to a comprehensive vision of affordable, accessible, and acceptable care for all.[1]

The ambition enshrined in the United Nation's Sustainable Development Goals of achieving UHC by 2030 has energized many governments to devise bold strategies and make big investments in their health systems. I have seen first-hand how the Philippines, Vietnam, Kenya, India, Indonesia, Columbia, Costa Rica, Panama, Nigeria, South Africa, Cyprus, islands across the Caribbean, and many others have announced significant UHC reforms since the development goals were passed in 2014, and UHC has been a headline issue in a number of national elections.

However, although UHC is proving a catalyst for change, the importance of the health workforce in achieving it is often hidden. Much of the debate focusses on financing systems—and national health insurance systems in particular—as a means to quickly and visibly 'cover' large sections of the population with increased access and entitlements. While increasing pooled financing for health is an essential step on the road to UHC, it is of limited value if used in isolation from delivery system reforms.[2] A new tax to fund health insurance can be levied and implemented within a year or two, but expanding the workforce to fulfil these new entitlements might take a decade or more. This asymmetry can create several perverse and damaging effects. Sadly, I have worked in many countries which spent a disproportion amount of time and effort thinking more about finance than people.

A global bidding war for talent

A key differentiator between the most and least successful UHC stories of the last decade is whether the financing and workforce components of reform are synchronized. While Mexico's Seguro Popular (popular insurance) programme was a major step forward in the country's progress towards UHC, it suffered from an overemphasis on health financing at the expense of delivery. The population of covered citizens nearly doubled over the first decade (from 51% in 2002 to 91% in 2014), while the supply of available hospital beds only increased by 13%, nurses 30%, and doctors 50%.[3,4] As a result, the drastic decrease in inequalities in insurance coverage did not lead to a similar impact on inequalities in access to key services or out-of-pocket health spending.[5]

Compare this with Thailand, which is frequently hailed as the benchmark of rapid UHC progress.[6] At the same time as its Universal Coverage Scheme was being established from 2001, huge investment in the capacity of the training system doubled the ratio of doctors and nurses per head of population over 15 years.[7] Key components of their strategy were new nursing and medical colleges, expansion of the existing institutions and recruitment of students from underserved communities, who they predicted would be less likely to emigrate. This was coupled with enlargement of Thailand's Village Health Volunteers scheme to more than one million mostly rural, female community health workers.

The danger is that if countries pursuing UHC choose short-term, politically visible strategies over long-term reform, much of the public resource now being invested by governments will be poured into a reactive bidding war for global talent rather than expanding access. With demand increasing faster than supply, health systems will attempt to outbid each other in attracting health workers, and wage rises will absorb money that could have gone towards additional capacity.

Romania is a recent example. After accession to the European Union more than 14,000 doctors, nurses, and midwives emigrated in search of higher salaries elsewhere in the continent.[8] In response, in March 2018 the government instituted dramatic salary rises—151–287% for resident doctors, 70–172% rises for nurses, and almost 400% for primary care doctors.[9,10] This will strain funding for the rest of the health system.

The losers of this global auction to raise salaries will, naturally, be poorer countries that are unable to compete on pay (see Fig. 18.1), especially given that many of the most active markets for health workers are currently Middle Eastern states that also offer low personal tax rates.

A welcome shift in global leadership

Fortunately, global leadership to highlight the workforce as a hidden dimension of UHC has been improving. The first years in the tenure of Dr Tedros Adhanom Ghebreyesus—the architect of Ethiopia's 'health worker flooding'[11] strategy of the early 2000s when he was health minister—as director general of the World Health Organization have been an important milestone.

He said: 'If we are to accelerate progress towards health for all, we must ensure that all people have equitable access to health workers . . . Almost half of the resources needed for achieving the health targets in the Sustainable Development Goals are related to the education and employment of health workers. This is not a cost to be contained; it's an investment to be nurtured. The fact is, investing in health workers creates jobs, drives inclusive economic growth, and increases productivity by getting sick people out of care and back to work.'[12]

But major gaps in global leadership still exist. For example, the indicators by which the World Health Organization (WHO) measures countries' progress towards UHC currently include ratios of physicians, surgeons, and psychiatrists per capita but do not capture nurses, midwives, or other cadres.[13] This is despite WHO's own figures showing that doctors make up just 2.6 million of the 18 million global shortage of health workers.

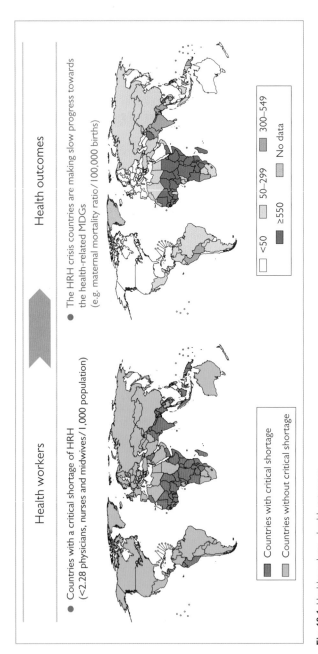

Fig. 18.1 Health workers—health outcomes.

Reproduced with permission from Siyam, A. (2014) Health Workforce Migration: A Roundtrip. Madrid, Spain: World Health Organization. Copyright 2014 WHO. Available at https://www.slideserve.com/elsa/health-workforce-migration-a-roundtrip-circulo-de-bellas-artes

There is a dearth of bold, creative ideas among global institutions on what to do about the health workforce crisis. While statements and frameworks to help countries prioritize their labour policies are helpful, their track record at driving change is poor. Among them is the Kampala Declaration, signed in 2008, which identified six pillars for a comprehensive health workforce such as national and global leadership, scaling up education and training, and managing the pressures of the international workforce market.

In the same way that the Millennium Development Goals inspired market-shifting initiatives such as the global vaccine alliance GAVI and the Global Fund to Fight AIDS, Tuberculosis and Malaria (which has dispersed more than US$30 billion so far) achieving UHC requires collaborations of scale and vision. What might such initiatives look like? Two of the most potent ideas I have come across are for a global medical university for low- and middle-income countries, and for investment in a number of countries as mass-production hubs exporting health workers to the world.

A global medical university

Perhaps the most revolutionary idea has been put forward by Dr Devi Shetty, founder of the Narayana Health chain in India—a pioneer of low-cost, high-quality surgery, often dubbed the Henry Ford of healthcare. He has proposed a global medical university that would do for education what he has already done for hospitals—standardize, achieve mass scale, and reduce the price.[14]

The idea challenges many of the cornerstones of classical medical education. Comprehensive seven-year degrees in general medicine would be replaced by immediate specialization in broad categories such as medicine, surgery, gynaecology, and paediatrics. In-person lectures by a local faculty would be replaced with interactive online teaching by the world's best medical teachers. Not touching a patient until years into study would be replaced by working as nurse auxiliaries on wards from day one.

As Dr Shetty describes: 'In the first month, the students will attend virtual dissection classes online. After this they will work in the hospital for five hours every day as nurse assistants and spend two hours a day in group discussions on anatomy, physiology, and biochemistry. In the second year, they can work as student doctors under medical specialists by taking care of the patients under the resident doctors. They will be substitutes for some of the activities performed by the nurses and also take part in on-call duty at night working as assistants to on-call doctors.'[15] The resulting degrees would be immediately transferrable to other member countries, which would allow global mobility without draining staff to high-income countries.

Under the current way of working, India needs 500 new medical colleges to secure enough doctors, each requiring an average set-up cost of US$50 million. Dr Shetty estimates that a global medical university run along the radical lines he proposes could establish 10,000 new colleges across Asia, Africa, and Latin America within a few years training up to 30,000 doctors every year.

Health workers as an economic export

Another transformative idea would be to invest in a small number of countries as global hubs for health worker training. While the unplanned export of health workers has undoubtedly had catastrophic effects on many health systems, more recent research has highlighted some of the benefits.[16] This shift from 'brain drain' to 'brain circulation' draws attention to the opportunities for skills transfer and remittance flows from skilled health workers going overseas.

The country that has famously taken advantage of health workers as an economic export is Cuba, which generates an estimated US$8 billion in revenues each year through more than 37,000 doctors and nurses it has working in around 77 countries.[17] Going out in teams or 'brigades' typically on three-year rotations, Cuba makes its health workers available in their thousands in exchange for a variety of benefits such as oil in the case of Venezuela and cash with richer African states such as Botswana and Kenya. They are often deployed for humanitarian and foreign policy reasons too, such as the Ebola crisis in West Africa and hurricanes Irma and Maria across the Caribbean.

Perhaps Cuba's most famous medical export initiative has been the 'Mais Medicos' (More Doctors) programme in Brazil.[18] Facing great difficulties recruiting primary healthcare workers into Brazil's remote and rural areas, 11,000 Cuban doctors were recruited to work across more than 4,000 underserved municipalities from 2016, treating an estimated 63 million people. It is believed that only around 25% of these workers' salaries were paid directly to them, with the remaining 75% going to the Cuban government. Sadly, as I describe in the next chapter, a political dispute is now unravelling this programme and the doctors have been heading back home.

Although Cuba's story is fascinating, an island of 12 million people can only make so big a dent in the global workforce gap. But what if countries such as India and the Philippines began to see it as an economic opportunity, and sought investment to achieve it?

Like Cuba, this could involve selling medical education and exporting trained staff. Taking the idea further, though, it could also mean exporting e-health services without people having to emigrate. India and the Philippines are already two of the largest call centre and outsourcing hubs in the world; what value could these capabilities create if directed towards providing global digital healthcare services?

The Philippines has already created a structural oversupply of nurses to mitigate the intense demand from the United States, Europe, and Middle East. The number of nursing colleges has increased from 170 in the 1990s to almost 500 today.[19] The 19,000 nurses that leave the Philippines every year send back billions of pesos annually, an important component in the remittance flows which make up around 10% of the country's GDP.[20]

With the exception of recent agreements with Japan, much of the health worker exodus from the Philippines is unplanned, and there is no doubt that this has been difficult for the health system to manage. Most perverse have been the effects of international barriers to Filipino doctors migrating abroad, which have led many to retrain as nurses in order to move. This is a lose-lose for all parties involved—yet there are now 45 colleges in the Philippines providing abridged courses for doctors to convert to nursing.[21] This should not deter bold thinking about the possibilities of global investment in intentional, and planned, exporting of health workers.

Low- and middle-income countries face three key challenges in building and retaining their workforce: finding creative ways to retain health workers and attract them back; escaping Western systems of professional regulation; and building a more constructive relationship with the private sector.

Creative ways to retain health workers and attract them back

Since low- and middle-income countries will never win in the global bidding war for health talent, they need to find more creative ways to retain the people they have and attract back workers who have left. While money is obviously a factor behind health worker emigration, safety, security, respect, dignity, and a sense of purpose and progression are just as important.[22]

This poignant quote from a migrating Kenyan doctor illustrates what can drive talent abroad: 'I can't quite decide if it is the night I performed two Caesarean sections with the anaesthetist shining the light from his mobile phone because the generator did not function . . . Or maybe it is the fact that over 60% of nurses in Southern Africa are HIV positive because of a lack of gloves. Or maybe it is the incidents of nurses being raped in night-time hours, sometimes by patients.'[23]

'Stick' approaches such as 'pay it back if you don't come back' training contracts and mandatory rural rotations for staff are helpful, but they will never be sufficient to combat powerful push factors such as poor working conditions.

As the primary beneficiaries of health worker migration, high-income countries have a duty to lead the effort to attract them back home. Even after international agreements to restrict flows from the poorest nations, high-income countries still sit at the top of a pipeline that draws labour from middle-income systems, and from low to middle in turn.

There are some commendable efforts. The UK's Department for International Development invests tens of millions of dollars each year in programmes to train health workers in Africa, but at the same time it is estimated that more than US$2 billion has been extracted from African countries in training doctors who subsequently leave.[24] The African Union estimates that rates of doctor emigration in Mozambique, Angola, and Malawi currently stand at 75%, 70%, and 59%, respectively.[25] This warrants considerable recompense.

Escaping Western systems of professional regulation

One area that exposes a dearth of innovation is how UHC-aspiring countries regulate health workers. From doctors to nurses to support staff, the majority of their professional regulation systems mirror those of the West. This creates administrative burdens that these systems are less equipped to absorb and locks in professional silos that increasingly do not make sense even in the West, let alone for far less well-resourced environments.

Dr Shetty of Narayana Health again gives a compelling perspective from India:

'The regulations that [India] has for medical healthcare are exactly how they are in the United States. We have a medical council (Indian Medical Association), which is an elected body that regulates our ethics and delivery. We are no different, but in the United States or in Europe, a doctor works for 48 hours a week. In India, doctors work for 48 hours a day. Yesterday I did three heart operations, saw 75 patients in my [out-patient department]. If I don't see that many patients, the next day I will have to see 200 of them.

'Statistically, 14 to 15% of pregnant women need a Caesarean section. That means we need to do nearly 5.2 million Caesarean sections per year. To do that, we need 200,000 gynaecologists; we have 50,000 of them . . . We need 200,000 anaesthetists; we have less than 50,000. We need 200,000 paediatricians; again we have less than 50,000 . . . All this has nothing to do with money . . . This country requires the liberation of nursing and paramedical education. That's all.'[26]

Building a more constructive relationship with the private sector

In many low- and middle-income countries in which I have worked the private sector is viewed, often with justification, as having a parasitic relationship with the healthcare workforce. They invest little in training but are happy to take the best skills from the labour pool that the public sector has developed. However, a recent survey of the 20 largest private healthcare provider chains in emerging markets found a significant proportion intend to change their business and service delivery models towards delivering UHC (Fig. 18.2).

There is clearly more that for-profit healthcare providers and educational institutions can do to develop the workforce needed for UHC. The lack of private sector voices in the global workforce debate at national and international levels is a missed opportunity to bring new ideas, capacity, and investment to finding solutions.

Looking at the role of the private sector in developing health systems, Imperial College London, and the CDC Group (a development finance institution owned by the UK government) proposed that private providers should 'put in more than they take out' in skills development.[27] The international hospital and clinic chain IHH Healthcare, which operates in 10 countries, is a good example of one such organization. Unlike many providers that claim to have developed a comprehensive care service, IHH incorporates medical education in its core activities. This includes three large teaching institutions allied to their largest facilities, including Malaysia's first private medical college, the International Medical University, and the Parkway College of Nursing and Allied Health in Singapore.

The scope for greater public–private partnerships in healthcare education and training is significant. However, the recent experience of Sri Lanka exposes the potential pitfalls if these agreements are not handled carefully. The South Asia Institute of Technology and Medicine (SAITM) was envisaged as a solution to the deadlock in Sri Lanka's current model of medical training. Free university education meant open access based on ability but, as a result of limited public funds, there were only

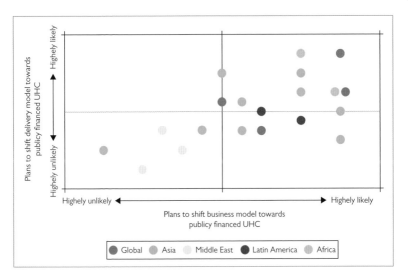

Fig. 18.2 Expectations of multinational private providers to change their business models in response to UHC.

Reproduced with permission from Qatar Foundation: Healthy returns—the role of private providers in delivering universal health coverage, 2018.

enough places for 17% of students that achieve the required grades.[28] This was far fewer than the health system needed.

Using private investment, SAITM was set up in 2013 to offer medical degrees. The institute faced relentless opposition from the medical community, who felt its high fees undermined the values of their profession. Doubts were also raised about the quality its medical education, leading the UK's General Medical Council to refuse recognition of SAITM degrees for further professional exams in Britain.[29] The institute acknowledged some of these criticisms, but also pointed out that the same level of scrutiny had never been applied to Sri Lanka's existing public medical schemes.

The end result was an ugly 'lose-lose' for all involved. In October 2017, the medical faculty of SAITM was closed and around 1,000 students faced an uncertain future, despite commitments to absorb them into other institutions.[30] No doubt SAITM's backers will be wary about future investments in the sector and the crisis has left a legacy of mistrust between policymakers and doctors.

A more positive example is one of Malaysia's longest standing public-private partnerships, the Melaka-Manipal Medical College.[31] For decades, thousands of Malaysian doctors were trained in India at what is now Manipal University, but this came to an abrupt end in 1993 when the Indian government introduced a policy preventing foreign medical students from training there. This created a shortage of opportunities for Malaysian medical students, leading to the MMMC joint venture.

In a deal signed that same year between the medical college and Manipal University, backed by both governments, students study medical degrees over five years, with time spent in both India and Malaysia. Over 300 medical students graduate annually, making the college the largest contributor of doctors to the Malaysian healthcare system.

Migrating ideas

Western countries have much to answer for in how they have shifted the burden of staff shortages to other nations, but it may be in years to come that ideas and innovations from less wealthy health systems also migrate from low to high income countries. One example of such an innovation that is already at work is Tonic in Bangladesh—a so-called 'digital front door to health for all' devised by one of the world's largest telecommunications companies, Telenor Health.

Working through Grameen Phone as distributor, Tonic was created as a free, value-adding service to the company's network subscribers. It offers 24/7 access to a medical helpline, which is supported by artificial intelligence and standardized medical protocols, a provider navigation system to help patients find the best place to seek care, 30% discounts at more than 800 enlisted providers, and a 'hospicash' micro-insurance benefit in the event of a hospitalization. Crucially, the product also communicates personalized healthcare content after patients interact with the system, helping to inform and motivate patients to maintain their health with minimal human input.[32]

Blending the telecoms company's consumer insights on how to build engagement and trust with world-class treatment protocols and healthcare information, Tonic provides a model for many other countries in empowering patients and delivering healthcare in new ways.

The ultimate prize

Our progress towards the goal of universal health coverage will be largely dependent on our collective willingness to face the challenge of the global health workforce crisis. I think it is possible for all countries to develop universal healthcare and believe it will be one of humankind's most important achievements this century. But governments and both the public and private sectors in countries which have not yet achieved it need to increase levels of trust, transparency, expertise, and mutual accountability. The future well-being of their people and nation depends on it.

Chapter 19

Brazil—power to the people

Brazil is a beautiful country and I have travelled its length from the Amazon to the Iguazu Falls bordering Argentina and Paraguay. I have seen its people at their kindest and witnessed violence too. There is a cynical saying in Brazil that 'it is the country of the future and always will be', meaning it will never fulfil its potential. There is no doubt that the 'Car Wash' scandal into money laundering, bribery, and corruption has rocked civil society, and business, politics, and the country is going through profound changes. But the country's Sistema Ùnico de Saúde (SUS), its unified health system, and PSF, the family health programme, provide vital social cohesion, and demonstrate what can be achieved with limited resources. They need to be protected and championed during these difficult times.

One of the largest free universal health systems in the world

Thirty years ago, Brazil's health system was patchy and elitist, serving mainly the rich or unionized white-collar workers and neglecting the poorest—those living without access even to clean water, sewage, or housing. Today, the country's Sistema Ùnico de Saúde (SUS) is one of the largest free universal health systems in the world. Conceived of as the country emerged from a brutal 20-year dictatorship and ushered into being by the same political movement that delivered Brazil back its civil democracy, 79% of Brazil's population now rely solely on the SUS for health services.[1]

Scaling a health system to that size is a major feat, and while there may still be issues with the numbers, quality, and distribution of staff, the achievement to date deserves praise. What Brazil has demonstrated with its workforce is the art of the possible. Unfortunately, many of the tailwinds that helped strengthen its health workforce are turning, and while it has much to teach from its own recent experience, it also has much to learn if it is to manage future workforce challenges.

Upskilling and upscaling

To deliver its constitutional promise of health for all, the SUS needed to grow at scale and pace—and it did. In 1980 there were around 18,500 health centres but by 2005 that number had more than tripled to 62,500.[2]

The upscaling of Brazil's clinical workforce is impressive. In the 20 years that followed inception of the SUS in 1988, the health workforce grew rapidly, leading to an improved ratio of staff to population.[3] For example, the number of physicians per 1,000 population in 1990 was 1.12. Today it is 1.85.[4] There were auspicious growth spurts too. Between 1999 and 2005 the number of doctors increased by almost a quarter and the number of nurses doubled. Then between 2006 and 2007, in just one year, the density of nursing staff shot up again, from 0.24 per 1,000 population to 0.94, along with nurse technicians from 0.15 to 2.47 and nursing aides (known as community health workers) from 0.6 to 3.16.[5]

Such steep growth in the workforce was made possible by a decision to expand the country's training capacity rapidly. Within three decades of the revolution, the number of medical school courses in Brazil had almost trebled, primarily the result of a huge expansion in the number of private medical schools, which started to out-number federal institutions in the late 2000s.[6] Brazil's 319 technical colleges spanning the length and breadth of the country provided training capacity for the new nurses, nurse technicians, and nursing aides.[7] They also provided the means for existing staff to up-skill through a process of continuous professional development, facilitated by parallel changes to regulation and legislation.

In addition to expanding training places, the Ministry of Education attempted to align the content of undergraduate teaching courses more closely with the needs of the population through its Pro-Saúde (Pro-Health) programme. But despite recognition from the World Health Organization (WHO) and the World Federation of Medical Education for its 'courageous' efforts, the public has been more critical, particularly about the quality of doctors graduating from private medical schools and the government's apparent failure to regulate them appropriately. There is a widespread perception that the primary objective of such schools is to make profit, particularly galling when so many of them are publicly subsidized.

Family healthcare

Brazil's focus was on expanding access to primary care, which it did through its now famous Estratégia Saúde da Família, or family health programme (ESF). The unique and fixed staff structure of the Primary Health Team with one doctor, one nurse, and six community health workers in each municipality required a radical change to the ratios of professionals in training. Figure 19.1 shows the extraordinary growth in community health workers required in comparison with other groups. Today, more than 280,000[8] of them serve nearly 70% of Brazil's population.[9]

Investment in community health workers was one of the key factors enabling the ESF to spread as far and wide as it did. The staff take less time to train and cost less to train and employ. They provide basic primary care to families at home, report back on patients' health to the municipal healthcare teams, attempt to resolve low-level problems as a first line, refer more complex problems to nurses or doctors, and collect data. As the Commonwealth Fund explains: 'The program, which costs $50 per person per year, has lessened the pressure on more expensive care providers and led to significant improvements in clinical outcomes nationally—reducing hospitalizations and mortality and improving equity and access.'[10]

It could do more. Many are now calling for the service to be digitalized, with electronic patient records and handheld devices for community health workers. This

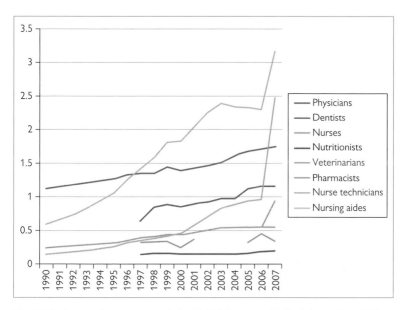

Fig. 19.1 Evaluation of human resources for health (HRH) ratios per 1,000 inhabitants, from 1990 to 2007, by occupation.

Reproduced from Buchan, J. et al. Continuity and change in human resources policies for health: lessons from Brazil. Human Resources for Health. 9(17). Copyright © 2011 Buchan et al.; licensee BioMed Central Ltd.

would be a great investment, and could go a long way to bridging the gaps between South and North and urban and rural and remote areas.

Mais Medicos

These huge improvements were not enough, and in 2013 the government could no longer ignore angry street protests about access to health services. First, although the health workforce had expanded, the distribution of staff was heavily skewed to more affluent states and cities in the South. Such inequality persists—compare the city of Vitoria with 11.9 physicians per 1,000 population with Macapá with just 1.41.[11] Second, although primary care had on the whole improved, there were significant shortages in some medical specialties such as paediatrics and anaesthetics and long waits for secondary care investigations and treatment. Government attempts to lure Brazilian doctors to needy municipalities by offering unusually high salaries or paying off student debts had failed because most doctors trained in public universities where no fees were chargeable and most medical students came from well-off families.

The Mais Medicos (more doctors) programme resulted from an agreement between the Brazilian government and the Pan American Health Organization (PAHO) that Brazil could recruit doctors from the PAHO region to work for up to three years in understaffed primary care teams before being repatriated and replaced. The plan worked. Before it started, 701 municipalities out of about 5,000 had no doctor. By 2018, not a single municipality was without one. According to independent evaluation, 94% of users report satisfaction with the doctors, 86% report that care quality has improved, and in some places waiting times in clinics declined 89% despite an increase of 33% in the average number of clinic and home visits each month.[12]

In 2018 however, the Mais Medicos programme took a huge blow. In response to comments from Brazil's President-elect, Jair Bolsonaro, the Cuban Government announced the withdrawal of all 8000 of its doctors from the scheme—half of the 16,000 total. Overnight, the care of 28 million people was threatened—around a hundred cities rely completely on Mais Medicos doctors for care.

Bolsonaro announced plans for doctors trained abroad to have their medical qualifications validated before continuing to practise in Brazil—a populist sentiment that had been grumbling for some time in the country.[13] He also argued the doctors should be paid the full sum of their wages (75% of the doctors' wages are siphoned off to PAHO) and that doctors working in Brazil should have the right to bring their families with them and settle. It was all too much for Cuba.

Mais Medicos is not a perfect programme by any means, but despite its faults, it was an overwhelming force for good in helping to expand access to care for Brazil's poorest citizens. They will struggle to make up for this acute loss and I fear that those ordinary citizens will pay the price for it.

Secrets of success

Buchan et al. (2011) describe some of the secrets of Brazil's early workforce successes. They cite a parallel expansion in management capacity as critical to the success of Brazil's early workforce policies—not an outcome most doctors would have predicted. Brazil systematically professionalized the management of human resources for health (HRH) at state and municipal level, a turning point being the establishment of a body within the Ministry of Health dedicated to strategic planning of the health workforce, the Secretariat of Labor and Education Management in Health. These planners worked behind the scenes to improve working conditions, update regulation of careers and salaries, and improve workforce mobility. They produced strategic guidelines for expanding the SUS and developed a comprehensive IT system designed to help model and plan the health labour market in Brazil.[14]

Managing expectations

For Brazil, like every other country promising universal health coverage, a growing demand for services is testing the limits of its love. Alongside economic growth and development, the last three decades have brought with them a tidal wave of obesity, diabetes, and other non-communicable diseases. Brazil's new middle class—the 36 million people to emerge from extreme poverty in a generation—are also becoming more demanding. Between 2010 and 2014, the number of medication lawsuits filed against the SUS increased 63%, most for contravening evidence-based guidelines set out in national protocols.[15] The Zika outbreak in 2015 put further pressure on an already overburdened service, and the economic downturn of 2014 hit health hard with a double whammy of increased numbers of citizens forced to rescind private medical insurance (many of them undergoing treatment) and reduced income from tax receipts. Even if it was possible to throw money at the workforce problem, the SUS doesn't have any. Constitutional Amendment 95, implemented in 2016, put a freeze on real terms growth in the healthcare budget for the following decade.[16]

There have been some admirable efforts to contain demand and Brazil can be proud of some of its successes. In the early 2000s Brazil famously leveraged the buying power of its huge health system to negotiate aggressively with multinational pharmaceutical companies on the cost of antiretroviral treatment, a policy that allowed the SUS to provide the drugs free of charge and prevented many AIDS deaths. The introduction of CONITEC, Brazil's answer to the UK's regulator National Institute for Health and Care Excellence (NICE), was also sensible, inevitable, and necessary for a free at the point of use universal health system.

The productivity puzzle

There is no hiding, however, that Brazil has to face its productivity problem head on. According to a report by Boston Consulting, for too long, Brazil has relied on increases in it working age population to drive economic growth. Between 2001 and 2013, for instance, only 22% of Brazil's gross domestic product (GDP) growth resulted from productivity gains. Contrast that with China and India, where 89% and 83%, respectively, came from growth in productivity.[17] The SUS is also inefficient. The World Bank reports that most Brazilian hospitals operate at a low level of efficiency (scoring an average 0.34 for technical efficiency on a scale of 0–1) due to small-scale operations, high staffing, and inefficient use of capacity and technology.[18] Many Brazilian hospitals may not even be capable of running efficiently—65% have fewer than 50 beds and occupancy rates run at about 37% for acute hospitals and 45% for all hospitals.[19] The traditional answer to this problem is consolidation, which is possible in more densely populated areas but harder in rural and remote ones like Amazonas.

Overzealous professional regulation stands in the way of increasing workforce productivity. Despite international evidence about the safety and efficacy of nurses taking on more advanced diagnosis and treatment, strong doctors' unions have opposed many such moves.

A tale of two Brazils

Brazil is a country of stark social and health inequalities. The South is richer, has better health infrastructure, and is still the place where most doctors and nurses want to live and work. The North lacks beds and X-ray machines, laboratories, and intensive care units. Entire clinics lack specialist providers such as paediatricians and the cost of transporting patients to clinics eats up large swathes of their budget.

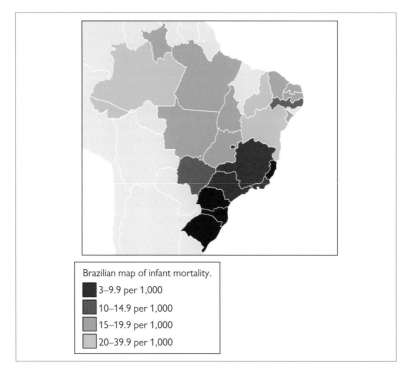

Fig. 19.2 Brazilian map of infant mortality.

Reproduced from Wikipedia. List of Brazilian states by infant mortality. Available at https://en.wikipedia.org/wiki/List_of_Brazilian_states_by_infant_mortality. Copyright © 2017 Wikipedia.

Outcomes suffer. For instance, the infant mortality rate is twice as high in the North as the South (Fig. 19.2).[20]

The potential for telehealth to bridge this yawning gap has not gone unnoticed. Never one to let the opportunity of creating a new governmental department pass it by, in 2016 Brazil set up the Permanent Telehealth Commission. Telehealth could help in two ways—facilitating more remote consultations and providing a means for clinicians to upskill through remote learning. By 2025, Latin America will have over 2.5 billion connected devices.[21] But current regulations only allow online consultations when a physician is present with the patient and another physician is consulted for second opinion. Overcoming challenges like this means facing down the powerful doctors' unions in Brazil, a challenge at such a fraught political time.

Conclusion

The SUS is a magnificent achievement and the workforce expansion that accompanied it a lesson to the world. Their family health programme delivered primary care at scale in large part by its focus on mobilizing huge numbers of community health workers. This is a great example of inverting the pyramid—investing in large numbers of lower-skilled staff rather than small numbers of medical specialists. Similarly, by massively increasing the number of nurses, they have increased the chances of getting good value out of their doctors. The success of the family programme can be seen in reductions in both infant mortality and admissions to hospital. Brazil's next challenge will be tackling the variations in quality, productivity, and distribution of its workforce.

But it will need to survive an extended period of austerity. After Brazil fell into recession in 2014 its government begun cutting public spending. According to the *British Medical Journal (BMJ)*, this hit the Bolsa Família (family allowance) programme, which pays families for vaccinating their children and keeping them in school. Infant mortality in Brazil rose for the first time in more than a quarter of a century in 2016. The Ministry of Health highlighted the zika virus, but there has been an increase in preventable infant deaths from diarrhoea and pneumonia alongside an increase in chronic malnutrition in the under-fives.[22] These are serious challenges. Let us hope that the words running through the Brazilian flag—Order and Progress—are made a reality for the mass of the population sometime soon.

Chapter 20

Conclusion—why some rabbits outrun foxes

Many years ago I heard a fable which I use quite a lot when travelling the world. It starts with a simple, benign question. Why do some rabbits outrun foxes? The answer is a little more poignant. For the rabbit, it is a question of life and death but for the fox it is merely a matter of lunch. It seems to me that workforce planning in health systems across the world has largely been seen as a question of ingestion not survival. All too often, like the Charles Dickens character Wilkins Micawber, the approach seems to be that 'something will turn up'. We need greater urgency to tackle this issue in a much broader context. If we do so I believe we have a good chance of increasing the capacity to care provided by the global health workforce by 20% by 2030.

We are in trouble

The central argument of this book is that over the next decade we are heading towards a global workforce shortage in healthcare that will harm patients, citizens, and societies. Knowing what we know we cannot simply watch this happen, and I believe it is possible to make good this gap by orchestrating our policies and practice in a more innovative, concerted, and collaborative way. In doing so, productivity will improve in a key section of the economy and national wealth will increase, helping individual prosperity, families, communities, and social cohesion.

I do not underestimate how difficult this is—it requires nothing less than the total reimagination of how we do things. It will involve the determined and careful coordination of many different agencies, institutions, and organizations which, left to their own uncoordinated and fragmented efforts, will fail because the size of the challenge transcends any normal linear solution. Solving the global workforce crisis in healthcare is a complex, wicked problem, but we can do better.

Five forces driving new approaches to care

I predict that by 2030 five forces will be driving radical change in the way we provide care. First, we will increasingly switch from face-to-face consultation to virtual channels facilitated by digital innovation and artificial intelligence.

Second, we will scale up primary care so it becomes the undisputed leader for promotion, prevention, and better population health management through sophisticated techniques for patient segmentation and stratification of need.

Third, from this primary and community care hub, patients and their carers will be supported to do more for themselves and with each other. This will include elderly care. Pharmacies will become wellness centres and places of support, training, and encouragement for patients and carers.

Fourth, standardized pathways and protocols for long-term conditions—supported by cognitive augmentation, digital communication, and artificial assistance—will form the basis of integrated pathways of care between hospitals and their referring physicians and clinicians. New integrated—or accountable—care organizations will become the norm.

Fifth, hospitals themselves will become Six Sigma centres of excellence known as high reliability organizations, driving patient quality, safety, and experience to new heights, reducing variation to only that which is clinically necessary. They will be supported by a vast array of digital solutions that include artificial intelligence (AI), robotics, cognitive augmentation, scheduling, rostering, and blockchain.

Based on these five dynamics, it is relatively straightforward to model, train, and supply the workforce of the future. Managing these five movements should improve productivity by 20%, releasing much needed capacity and time to care.

Of course, new therapeutic, diagnostic, and interventional techniques, treatments, and innovations will come along during the next decade, but they will not substantially disrupt the dominant approaches to care. The paradox of today's healthcare is that its medicine is led by twenty-first century global thinking but its delivery is hindered by nineteenth-century cottage industry organization. I have high hopes for genomics and personalized medicine, but it will take time. We are safe to plan for different workforce roles over the next decade because that is at least how long it will take us to implement the five key movements described. Elements of all five exist across the world but have seldom been put together.

Productivity—health is wealth

In terms of how we respond to these five forces, I want to simplify and amplify some of the main points used in support of my argument. First, we need to reframe the workforce debate to one of national productivity. Healthcare already accounts for one-tenth of many economies and what it does—or does not do—matters substantially. To improve productivity in a growing sector of society requires long-term investment in education, training, skills, innovation, technology, infrastructure, research, management, and leadership, to name but a few. Governments patently cannot do all this by themselves from the centre, so a new, entrepreneurial state will need to generate public and private investment. I have yet to find any clear masterplan from my travels but I have seen some decent efforts—such as in Singapore—which attempt to harness the power of different stakeholders.

Governments not only have a legitimate convening role but one of active shaping as well. Their central responsibility is to ensure health services are satisfactorily resourced so that demand is manageable and the workforce supply is abundant. In Organisation for Economic Co-operation and Development (OECD) countries, the share of population aged 65 years and older increased from 12% in 1990 to 16% in 2015 and is expected to grow to 21% in 2030 and 27% in 2050.[1] Facing similar problems, Singapore has a thoughtful approach to its workforce strategy based around three pillars—jobs and skills, productivity, and innovation. For jobs, they provide multiple pathways to attract mid-career locals to enter healthcare and are redesigning jobs and enhancing skills to support a 'future-ready workforce'. For productivity, they are streamlining workflows to focus on patient care and reduce non-value adding tasks. They are also investing at scale in assistive equipment and cost-effective technologies to lighten work, especially for older workers. For innovation, they are using technology to empower patients to care more for themselves, and have developed an impressive electronic health record connecting every provider. They would not claim to have thought through every policy lever and still have traditional 'doctor and patient' relationships—as well as doctors to every other clinician—but their planning horizon and timeframe are good.

Government should shape

We have also seen that governments across the world are doing more to address supply. Traditional 'pool and flow' models of supply and demand are too static and rigid to deliver all the necessary staff. In various parts of the world, action is now being taken on a number of uncoordinated fronts which would be more impactful if orchestrated together. Extending pensionable working ages is fair given increased life expectancy, while some countries extend working hours judiciously. We have seen the promotion of health jobs in countries such as Norway, which has nearly 20% of its working population in the sector[2] compared with Greece, which stands at just over 5%.[3]

Female participation rates in health employment are highly variable across the OECD and a move to normalize towards Northern European rates of female participation would, in itself, deliver a 10% increase in supply.[4] Further, in education and regulation policies, governments can change the rules of the game that are stacked towards an undersupply of clinical professionals. The relaxation of *numerus clausus* policies coupled with a regulatory environment that encourages and facilitates new models of care would all improve labour availability and workforce productivity.

New models of care are often talked about as a complicating factor in workforce planning. Proponents of this argument claim that clinical services, science, genomics, technology, and consumer power are changing too rapidly to predict the health workforce needs of society accurately over a decade. They are right to think it is all but impossible to precisely compute the specific number of psychiatrists, physicians, surgeons, interventional radiologists, advanced nurse practitioners, and allied health workers that will be needed. But they are wrong to conclude that we do not know what the prevailing approaches to care will be in 10 years' time. The paradox of healthcare is that scientific change can happen quickly, but change across systems can evolve all too slowly. For example, great advances in telehealth and smartphone technology have yet to disrupt the outpatient clinic, itself a construction of the eighteenth century which helped doctors not to walk too far from their hospital inpatient beds.

Patients as partners, communities as carers

Somewhat counter-intuitively, one of the five key movements will be to see patients and carers as an essential part of the workforce. Simply paying our taxes or health insurance will no longer be enough; we need to become active participants in our own care. Health systems need to promote this move for us to take greater responsibility for our own well-being.

KPMG member firms have contributed to an extensive body of literature that suggests patients can reduce consumption of services by 8% to 21% when they are empowered and supported to take more control of their care.[5] There are four levels of activation, and those patients that have been educated, trained, and supported (with real-time data, mobile applications, and peer-to-peer group assistance) to take care of various long-term conditions report better experiences and outcomes. NESTA, the innovation foundation for the United Kingdom, published The Business Case for People Powered Health, an impressive report which illustrates the magnitude of the problem. People with long-term conditions account for 50% of all GP appointments, 65% of all outpatient visits, and 70% of all inpatient bed days. Through a five-pronged approach, NESTA claims patients reduce appointments, visits, and admissions by 7% and saw gains of up to 20% in some pilot sites.[6]

Germany, which has the highest proportion of people aged over 65 in Europe, historically had a fragmented social care system administered by local states. Sweeping changes created mandatory long-term care insurance which currently stands at 2.5% of wages, with half coming from the employer.[7] Eligibility is broadly determined by the level of care dependency or cognitive impairment and benefits are distributed in two ways: cash payments to the individual needing care who can choose to pay a family member, volunteer or paid carer; and in-kind professional services. Levels of benefits are based on dependency and currently range from approximately €400 to €1,800 per month.[8] Most beneficiaries receive home care, and studies have shown this is a less expensive and more welcome option for most. Imagine the enormous productive power of having patients as partners and communities as carers. No health system will be sustainable unless it embraces this movement urgently.

Professions at the top of their game

Of course, we will still need more health staff. We just don't need more of the same. We would be in a better position to assess real needs if we could empower patients and communities, demystify clinical pathways, and look at the tasks required to ensure we had the right care in the right place at the right time. We need clinical professionals and community care workers that practise at the top of their game, often working to the limits of their scope of practice.

There is evidence of a considerable skills mismatch which is wasting human capital. The OECD report 'Health Employment and Economic Growth: An Evidence Base' says that results from the Programme for the International Assessment of Adult Competencies (PIAAC) 'shows that a large proportion of doctors and nurses reported being overskilled or underskilled for some of the tasks they need to perform. Around 70% of doctors and 80% of nurses reported being overskilled for some aspects of their work, while about 50% of doctors and 40% of nurses reported being underskilled for other tasks'.[9] If this is true it suggests that many tasks and jobs are so badly designed that they are barely fit for purpose, dragging down productivity and causing frustration, stress, and burnout.

A more sober analysis of the tasks needed to care for patients over the next decade would strongly suggest a greater need for generalists and peripatetic community workers supported by cognitive assistance, artificial intelligence, and robotics. The tribal demarcations between health and social care (in the NHS there are over 300 job types[10]) must give way to clear pathway management which standardizes many tasks, enabling new sources of local labour to be employed. This is not an argument about dumbing down health professions. It is the reverse. Allowing professionals to work at the top of their game will reduce frustration, enhance career progression, and improve productivity. As medical specialists and generalists create room for medical assistants, nurses, and allied health advanced practitioners to use their full repertoire of skills, this will create space for a new cadre of care workers that move between the home, community, and hospital. Coupled with new digital technologies, the care and productivity gains would be enormous, while encouraging greater social mobility through local community employment.

Arms and legs, not bodies

Clearer analysis and modelling of tasks—not job descriptions—is the way other industries are developing superior workforce shaping and employee agility. They are less concerned with rigid demarcations between tribal staff groups and much more preoccupied with the digitally enabled tasks that need to be delivered to customers. Companies and their human resources (HR) departments are becoming increasingly affected by recent advances in computational power and AI and are developing visual tools and models that help them reshape tasks and roles to drive greater customer satisfaction and productivity. Naturally, people fear the rise of the robots because job losses could be significant.

I was a member of the World Economic Forum whose founder, Klaus Schwab, published *The Fourth Industrial Revolution*. It argues that the application of artificial intelligence to cognitive work and robotics to manual work will bring social and economic dislocation on a scale comparable to the original industrial revolution of the nineteenth century. Fears have been fuelled by books such as *Weapons of Math Destruction: How Big Data Increases Inequality and Threatens Democracy*. No doubt some fears are well placed, but I do not believe that health staff should feel threatened because, for the foreseeable future, demand will far outstrip supply.

Currently it is estimated that over the next decade automation will change every job category by at least 25%.[11] Often, however, these forecasts are made from fairly high-level surveys asking job holders what they do. It is far better to analyse role tasks and then evaluate what level of digital support can be adopted. Currently, only 5% of all occupations could be fully automated and it is important to remember the rather blunt phrase that AI 'rarely takes out bodies but can replace arms or legs', meaning that tasks can be replaced much more easily than eradicating a job. This is where healthcare has gone wrong. Fearing job losses and lacking the sophistication of task scheduling, layer upon layer of technology has been added to redundant, old-fashioned care and business processes.

Foo fighters

This is where tools and techniques such as *foo.castr* (future of organization caster) are crucially important. The KPMG Data Observatory developed with (and at) Imperial College in London analyses real tasks performed by staff which are then subject to data visualization techniques. This enables work teams and managers to confidently assess which tasks can be digitized and automated. The process rarely takes away whole jobs, but it dramatically shifts and shapes tasks so that new models can be imagined.

In healthcare, many organizations are sleepwalking into the future and there is little meaningful interplay between the educationalists, clinicians, managers, and technologists. Realizing the digital dividend takes a lot more preparation and detailed understanding of the tasks people perform. Of course, this challenge will become more acute because workforce management will no longer just be about labour supply and demand. Leaders will need to rethink the relationship between the organization, its technology, people, and the societies in which they operate. I am delighted to see that my old organization, University Hospitals Birmingham NHS Foundation Trust in the United Kingdom, is experimenting with *foo.castr* to learn and lead the way again.

The nature of work and organizations and their structure and leadership will need to change profoundly as digital disruption gathers momentum. It is the failure to get to grips with this which explains why change in healthcare is often poorly implemented and frustratingly slow. I have seen world class clinicians and clinical teams, in outstanding facilities, perform miracles with new technology. But I have yet to see the health sector harness the digital revolution at the scale and speed of other industries.

Nothing to fear but fear itself

If any industry has more to gain and less to fear from robotics, cognitive augmentation, digital disruption, and artificial intelligence, it is healthcare. The powerful combination of data and analytics is fuelling precision and personalized medicine and pushing genomics to new scientific frontiers. A recent review by American cardiologist Eric Topol on preparing the healthcare workforce to deliver the digital future illustrates the many shining but localized examples of what digital technology can achieve.[12] Topol argues that 'the real power of these technologies is likely to lie at their intersection. The fusion of genomics, digital medicine (including patient generated data) and AI could deliver a more holistic approach to personalized healthcare and disease prevention'.

He adds: 'Carefully designed AI algorithms will also enhance NHS productivity, through large scale process optimization, clinical pathway streamlining and public health applications. By offloading some human tasks to machines . . . clinical workflow and productivity could be greatly improved throughout the NHS.' What's not to like about this vision? Humans must learn to live in harmony with machines.

The hype around what AI can do—and what it can destroy—has not helped. I have had the opportunity of seeing many super-smart systems in Australia, Japan, China, Singapore, India, Israel, Germany, the United Kingdom, and the United States. I have yet to see their benefits fully materialize but neither have I seen the worst nightmares realized. Over time, these benefits will come. It is time humans took control and mobilized on a much grander scale.

Estimates suggest that, over the next 10 years, perhaps 60% of all jobs could have one-third of their tasks automated.[13] We already know what other industries are doing with administrative and clerical functions. NHS Digital estimates that the NHS employs 1.2 million people in England including 369,000 clinical support staff and a further 192,000 infrastructure and administrative support staff.[14] Digitization, automation, robotics, and blockchain could transform these services and dramatically enhance productivity. But action must be taken at scale to justify the upfront investment costs, and employment rights and education must be guaranteed for those who want to retrain.

There are enormous transaction costs between payers and providers in both socialized and (more so) private healthcare as contracts, bills, and money pass around the system. The same can be said for clinical information. Blockchain is already revolutionizing these types of transactions in other industries. With appropriate education, retraining, support, and encouragement, many staff could play a more prominent role in patient care. In the twenty-first century, we will not only need to be educated when we are young but when we are mid-career as well. Health systems are ideally placed to use this talent because they understand the high costs of recruiting new workers and exorbitant costs of agency contractors. Staff that emotionally commit to the values and purpose of a healthcare organisation are priceless.

Reimagining organizations and work

As technology changes jobs, roles, and tasks, so will the very nature of the organization itself. Organizational agility is the new, fashionable catchphrase. Some companies have sought to move away from a mechanical, rigid, bureaucratic hierarchy to a nimble, flexible, task-orientated enterprise which can adapt and change quickly to a volatile environment. Unlike traditional bureaucracies designed for stability and status, agile organizations offer dynamism and creativity. They typically refer to an interconnected network of teams (ironically, sometimes called chapters or guilds, reflecting the independence of some nineteenth-century workers) that work on task-and-finish projects to keep the organization evolving. Companies that have adopted this approach have seen a productivity boost. This is important for healthcare which is, generally speaking, hierarchical and bureaucratic. Without a change of leadership culture and organizational design, health organizations are going to find it hard to cope with the future.

That said, there is hope. Most clinical teams are semi-autonomous already and tend to collaborate for the immediate task at hand. Their innate desire to provide high-quality care needs to be harnessed to systems which better manage individual and team development, performance feedback, and design thinking, where they are clear what is expected of them and are supported in achieving it. It is impossible to change any organization if staff do not know what is expected of them, given the responsibility to get on with the job and then held to account. Professor Michael West and others have illuminated the fundamental relationship between a healthy organization, motivated clinical teams, and better patient care.[15]

In the corporate sector, the next generation of performance management systems appear to be aligned to a coaching approach. Employees are encouraged to be active in their learning and seek feedback to evaluate their progress and growth regularly, not just once a year. Increasingly, this approach allows teams to provide coaching and feedback to leaders which fosters a healthy and confident culture for change. These systems can improve productivity and help create more time to care.

Apperception

The more I researched for this book, the more I reflected on my 30 years' experience and concluded that the worldwide workforce crisis is what academics call a wicked problem, or what Harvard academic Robert Heifetz calls an 'adaptive challenge'. Adaptive problems are often systematic challenges with no ready answers. Descartes used the word 'apperception' to describe a process which allows leaders to use their cumulative experience to recognize patterns in situations that facilitate better understanding and thus possible resolution. Professor Keith Grint, of my alma mater, the University of Warwick, says apperception is 'the ability to frame or reframe situations so that what appeared to be one thing might actually be another or, more often, what appeared to be 'senseless' could be made sense of'. Although I'm no expert in management theory or French philosophy, the thinking behind these ideas chimes with my reflections and experience.

For adaptive challenges, Heifetz and others suggest that 'leaders do not need to know all the answers but they do need to ask the right questions' and go on to say that 'solutions to adaptive challenges reside not in the executive suite but in the collective intelligence of the employees at all levels who need to use one another as resources, often across boundaries, and learn their way to solutions'. This book is certainly asking questions and offering some ideas, but I hope its real purpose will be to get people talking, thinking, and acting differently together.

We know that around 75% of major change programmes fail, and the health industry is no stranger to periods of 're-disorganization'. One of the reasons for failure is that organizations and people apply erroneous and traditional management thinking to complex situations. For Grint, believing a situation or challenge to be a 'tame problem' when it is actually a complex, adaptive issue is a recipe for failure. Tame problems can sometimes be complicated and knotty but can be solved through technical management processes and skills. Wicked problems are not just complicated but complex, requiring a different way of thinking, acting, and mobilizing. They need distributed leadership, with authority passing from one to the many. Heifetz talks of six principles for leading adaptive work: 'Getting onto the balcony; identifying the adaptive challenge; regulating distress; maintaining disciplined attention; giving the work back to the people, and protecting voices of leadership from below.'

When I think of my years in healthcare, this model of change feels right for the workforce crisis. The traditional 'pool and flow' models built for workforce modelling are both deeply technical and deterministic. It is not that this work is wrong, but by itself it can never be right. Indeed, as some human resource professionals have said to me, it is not that workforce planning is wrong, it is that the design of models of care is badly thought through and executed.

As we have seen, the health workforce challenge is mirrored in demography, society, the economy, consumers, customers, patients, and technology, to name but a few. Put simply, it is too big a problem for a traditional national, regional, or local linear healthcare or workforce plan. However, politicians and others at local, state, or national level often feel this is their best remedy. As Heifetz forebodingly remarks, the 'prevailing notion that leadership consists of having a vision and aligning people with that vision is bankrupt because it continues to treat adaptive situations as if they were technical: the authority figure is supposed to divine where the company is going and people are supposed to follow'. This book is not trying to sell a solution. It is not a textbook or manual. It is just a book intended to make you think for yourself, while offering some ideas and strategies that seem to be working in different parts of the world.

Yes, we can

Surviving cancer has made me an even greater optimist about the future than before my radical prostatectomy. I am sure it is possible to create 20% greater capacity to care over the next decade, but only if we start thinking in a different way. Professor Richard Beckhard, one of the pioneers of organizational development, developed a formula for change that I learned 30 years ago when I was on the NHS Management Training Scheme: change is possible when A + B + C > D. A represents shared dissatisfaction with the current state of affairs; B the shared vision of the future state; C the collective commitment to the first practical steps; and D the resistance and opposition to change. Globally, in healthcare, we are currently stuck in 'A'.

This book is all about making change happen. I see, worldwide, dissatisfaction with the current state of affairs where rich countries rob poor ones of their clinical staff and powerful organizations outbid weak ones for talent. Yet even the winners of this perverse race do not have enough staff. Ultimately, it is a self-defeating game. Humans can do better than this. As a start, we need to work collectively and collaboratively on a better shared vision for our models of care and workforce needs. This requires all the right industries, organizations, and individuals to be in the same tent. Of course, there will not be a strict formula for success, but I would organize this at state or regional level because my observation is that health change is most meaningful with populations sized around five to eight million, as these are big enough to mobilize and leverage resources but small enough to maintain personal contact; think places like Singapore, Israel, and parts of the Nordics or the regions, provinces, or states of, respectively, England, Canada, Australia, and the United States. These places have an identity which is commonly recognized. At this macro level, I would involve public, private, community, and civil society leaders and organizations to start to discuss problems, explore possibilities, and sketch out solutions. In the same way that world-leading technology companies have powered out of San Francisco, Beijing, Shanghai, Bangalore, Singapore, Sydney, Berlin, Tel Aviv, and London, we need new clusters and networks of imagination and interest to solve this 'wicked problem'. We need to celebrate difference and exploit its potential.

At the meso or intermediate level—say a population base of between one and three million—we could create new joint venture partnerships between public, charitable, and private players. For example, technology is moving too fast to be controlled and shackled by the public sector but, fortunately, health expenditure is largely shaped by government action. Similarly, the health professions largely control education and training but families and communities provide the vast majority of care. I could go on, but the real point of this exercise would be to jointly commit to find solutions through partnerships forged through different experience and expertise.

At the micro or health system level, I would create test beds and taskforces which do the work. There is a fundamental problem with care model and workforce re-design, often referred to as the difference between 'work as imagined and work as done'. As there can be no room for confusion when professionals are caring for patients at the health system level, I would test whole systems with the key ideas suggested in this book along with the many other great examples of success found around the world. Health systems or organizations could test all or some, but networked or joint venture partnerships would lock in commitment and investment at scale over time.

These test beds would have regulatory freedom and permission to act and harness the best of public, non-government, and private expertise, resources, and intellectual property. They would be limited in number but grand in ambition and scale. Ironically, the old and outdated surgical concept of 'see one, do one, and teach one' might offer a model of spread across healthcare organizations. In my experience, this is how things are usually adopted and adapted in the health industry.

There is little merit in offering a neat, linear solution to the global workforce crisis, because life and change are messy. In the Preface I noted how the book cover was an altered image of Michelangelo's magnificent art. There is an old saying that 'God laughs when we make plans' but, somewhat divinely, humans can always move heaven and earth to find solutions when we really want to. It took Michelangelo four years to paint the Sistine Chapel, but we have a little longer. Let's get going.

Acknowledgements

I have been incredibly fortunate in building lasting friendships with work colleagues over the past 30 years of my career—that's one of the great things about healthcare. I would like to thank the people noted below who kindly offered me (in a personal capacity) advice and wise counsel.

International Review Panel

Dr Francisco Balestrin, President, International Hospital Federation (IHF) Geneva, Switzerland; President of the Brazilian College of Healthcare Executives

Professor David Bloom, Economics and Demography, Harvard School of Public Health, Harvard University, United States of America

Ms Anita Charlesworth CBE, Director of Research and Economics, Health Foundation, London

Lord Nigel Crisp, former CEO of NHS and Permanent Secretary of the Department of Health (2000–2006) and Global Chair, *Nursing Now*

Professor Nigel Edwards, CEO, Nuffield Trust, London, United Kingdom

Mr David Flory CBE, Chief of Tertiary Hospitals, Hamad Medical Corporation, State of Qatar

Professor Detlev Ganten, President, World Health Summit and former CEO, Charite, Berlin, Germany

Ms Elizabeth Koff, Secretary for Health, New South Wales, Australia

Professor Ling Li, Health Economics, Peking University, China

Sir Jonathan Michael, former CEO, Oxford University Hospitals, Guy's and St Thomas' Hospital, and University Hospitals Birmingham, United Kingdom

Sir Robert Naylor, Non-executive Director, Cleveland Clinic, Abu Dhabi and former CEO University College Hospital, London

Sir David Nicholson, former CEO of the NHS (2006–2014) and Visiting Professor of Global Health Innovation, Imperial College, London

Dr Patricia Oakley, Workforce Research Fellow, Kings College London, United Kingdom

Ms Sangita Reddy, Managing Director, Apollo Hospital Group, India

Professor Kevin Smith, President and CEO, University Health Network, Toronto, Canada;

Dr Yasuhiro Suzuki, Vice Minister for Health, Chief Medical and Global Health Officer, Ministry of Health, Labour and Welfare, Government of Japan

Specialist opinions

Mr David Amos, former Deputy Human Resources Director for the NHS, Department of Health, United Kingdom

Dame Ruth Carnall, Chair, Carnall-Farrar Management Consultancy, London, United Kingdom

Mr Simon St-Clair Carter, Consultant Urologist and former Medical Director, The London Clinic, United Kingdom

Professor Paul Corrigan CBE, former Special Advisor to Prime Minister, United Kingdom

Professor Ian Cumming, CEO, Health Education England, United Kingdom

Mr Bob Dearden, Founder, Dearden Consulting (retired), United Kingdom

Ms Pam Garside, Fellow, Judge Business School, University of Cambridge, United Kingdom

Ms Mary Jo Haddad, former President and CEO, SickKids, Toronto, Ontario, Canada

Sir Chris Ham, former CEO, King's Fund, London, United Kingdom

Ms Samantha Jones, CEO, Centene UK, United Kingdom

Mr Tim Jones, Director of Workforce and Innovation, University Hospitals Birmingham, West Midlands, United Kingdom

Mr Peter Lees, CEO and Medical Director, Faculty of Medical Leadership and Management, United Kingdom

Mr Roy Lilley, Health Commentator and Founder, Academy of Fabulous Stuff, United Kingdom

Ms Karen Lynas, former Managing Director of NHS Leadership Academy and KPMG Associate, United Kingdom

Professor Karen Middleton CBE, CEO, Chartered Society of Physiotherapy, United Kingdom

Ms Rebecca Myers, Community Nurse and Organisational Development Specialist, United Kingdom

Ms Kavita Narayan, Technical Advisor for Health and Skills at the Ministry of Health and Family Welfare, Government of India

Mr Dean Royles, former Director of Human Resources, Leeds Teaching Hospitals, United Kingdom

Dr Keith Ruddle, Associate Fellow, Said Business School, University of Oxford, United Kingdom

Dr Masami Sakoi, Director, Medical Economics Division, Health Insurance Bureau, Ministry of Health, Labour and Welfare, Government of Japan

Mr Shane Solomon, former CEO of the Hong Kong Hospital Authority and Managing Director of Telstra Health, Australia

KPMG team

Dr Edward Fitzgerald, Global Healthcare Practice Executive, KPMG International, and former surgeon

Ms Shubhangi Gupta, Team Leader, Global Clients and Research, Healthcare and Life Sciences, KPMG Global Services

Dr Charlotte Refsum, Global Healthcare Practice Executive, KPMG International, and General Practitioner

Mr Jonty Roland, Program Director, Center for UHC, KPMG International

Dr Aizhan Tursunbayeva, Senior Project Consultant, KPMG Italy

Mr Richard Vize, Director, Public Policy Media, United Kingdom

Notes

Preface: Cognitive dissonance

1. Dublin Declaration on Human Resources for Health (2017)
2. Liu et al., Global Health Workforce Labor Market Projections for 2030, Human Resources for Health (2017)

Chapter 1

1. Liu et al., Global Health Workforce Labor Market Projections for 2030 (Human Resources for Health, 2017)
2. Cometto G, Health workforce needs, demand and shortages to 2030: an overview of forecasted trends in the global health labour market, *UN High Level Commission on Health Employment and Economic Growth* (WHO, 2016)
3. World Health Organization statistics, Life expectancy at birth (WHO, 2014)
4. Institute for Health Metrics and Evaluation, Life expectancy at birth (IHME, 2014)
5. World Health Organization—Global Health Workforce Alliance, A universal truth: no health without a workforce (WHO, 2014)
6. Wu Q, Zhao L, & Ye X, Shortage of healthcare professionals in China, *The British Medical Journal*, 354, i4860 (2016)
7. Global health care outlook: common goals, competing priorities (Deloitte, 2015)
8. Aoki M, Nursing care workers hard to find but in demand in aging Japan (*The Japan Times*, 27 June 2016)
9. Bureau of Labor Statistics, Occupational employment projections: registered nurses (BLS, 2014)
10. Knickman JR & Snell EK, The 2030 problem: caring for aging baby boomers, *Health Services Research*, 37(4), 849–84 (2002)
11. Haddad LM & Toney-Butler TJ, *Nursing Shortage* (StatPearls Publishing, 2018)
12. AMN healthcare survey
13. Association of American Medical Colleges, The complexities of physician supply and demand: projections from 2016 to 2030 (AAMA, 2018)
14. Taylor H, Who is the world's biggest employer? The answer might not be what you expect (World Economic Forum, 17 June 2015)
15. *The Guardian*, 20 June 2017
16. Kentish B, How reliant is the NHS on foreign doctors? (*Independent*, 4 June 2018)
17. GCC total population 2010–2015. Gulf labour markets and migration, November 2016
18. Organisation for Economic Co-operation and Development, Foreign-trained doctors and nurses (OECD, 2017)
19. Deloitte, Time to care: securing a future for the hospital workforce in Europe (Deloitte, 2017)

20. Organisation for Economic Co-operation and Development, Foreign-trained doctors and nurses (OECD, 2017)

21. World Health Organization, Migration of health workers—WHO code of practice and the global economic crisis, 2014

22. Ibid.

23. Blacklock C, Heneghan C, Mant D, & Ward AM, Effect of UK policy on medical migration: a time series analysis of physician registration data, *Human Resources for Health*, 10, 35 (2012)

24. Nair M & Webster P, Health professionals' migration in emerging market economies: patterns, causes and possible solutions, *Journal of Public Health*, 35(1), 157–63 (2013)

25. Waldmeir P, China's doctors not part of society's elite (*Financial Times*, 6 October 2013)

26. Vidal P, The emigration of health-care workers: Malawi's recurring challenges (Migration Policy Institute, 21 October 2015)

27. Ibid.

28. WHO Global Code of Practice on the International Recruitment of Health Personnel, 2010

29. Tam V, Edge JS, & Hoffman SJ, Empirically evaluating the WHO global code of practice on the international recruitment of health personnel's impact on four high-income countries four years after adoption, *Globalization and Health*, 12, 62 (2016)

30. Office of National Statistics, Public service productivity estimates for healthcare (ONS, 2015)

31. Australian Productivity Commission, Increasing Australia's future prosperity (Productivity Commission, 2016)

Chapter 2

1. Krugman PR, The age of diminished expectations: U.S. economic policy in the 1990s, MIT Press (1990)

2. European Commission, European Policy Brief: output and productivity growth in the healthcare sector: a study of four European countries (European Commission, 2013)

3. Bojke C, Castelli A, Grašic K, Howdon D, & Street A, Productivity of the English NHS: 2013/14 Update, Centre for Health Economics, University of York (2016). https://www.ons.gov.uk/economy/economicoutputandproductivity/publicservicesproductivity/articles/publicservicesproductivityestimateshealthcare/financialyearending2017

4. New Zealand Productivity Commission, Understanding Health Sector Productivity, December 2017

5. The Government of UK, Policy paper Autumn Budget 2017, 22 November 2017

6. Jamison et al., Global health 2035: a world converging within a generation, *The Lancet*, 382(9908), 1898–955 (2013)

7. Bloom DE, Canning D, & Sevilla J, The effect of health on economic growth: a production function approach, *World Development*, 32, 1–13 (2004).

8. Robyn S, Cancer and economic growth in an aging population: estimating the impact for Australia (discussion paper, Griffith University, 2010)

9. Addicott et al., Workforce planning in the NHS (King's Fund, 2015)

10. Licchetta M & Stelmach M, *Fiscal Sustainability and Public Spending on Health*, Office for Budget Responsibility (2016)

11. Monitor, Helping NHS providers improve productivity in elective care (Monitor, 2015)

12. Organisation for Economic Co-operation and Development, The future of productivity (OECD, 2015)

13. Collins B, Adoption and spread of innovation in the NHS (The King's Fund, 16 January 2018)

14. Unlocking productivity through healthcare delivery innovations (McKinsey & Co, January 2010)

Chapter 3

1. World Health Organization, The health workforce in India, Human Resources for Health Observer Series No. 16 (2016)

2. World Bank Statistics, Physicians (per 1,000 people) (2016)

3. Govindarajan V & Ramamurti R, Delivering world class care affordably: In: *Harvard Business Review* (2013)

4. Ibid.

Chapter 4

1. World Health Organization, Israel health profile (WHO, 2014)

2. Pyutrikovsky S, Israel's doctor shortage (*Israel National News*, 21 December 2016)

3. Linder-Ganz R, More medical students in Israel won't help if there are no jobs available (Haaretz, 23 July 2018)

4. Linder-Ganz R, Israelis turned down for medical school to make room for foreigners (Haaretz, 10 July 2018)

5. Linder-Ganz R, More medical students in Israel won't help if there are no jobs available (Haaretz, 23 July 2018)

6. Israeli Medical Association, *The Physician Shortage in Israel*: Chapter 1: Background—the crisis in the healthcare system (Israeli Medical Association, 2018)

7. Horowitz PK, Shemesh AA, & Horev T, Is there a doctor in the house? Availability of Israeli physicians to the workforce, *Israel Journal of Health Policy Research*, 6(31) (2017)

8. OECD, Health at a glance, 2017

9. Siegel-Itzkovich J, Shortage of nurses in neonatal units leads to infant fatalities (*The Jerusalem Post*, 24 November 2015)

10. Siegel-Itzkovich J, French immigrant nurses protest against red tape in government (*The Jerusalem Post*, 21 August 2017)

11. Winer S, Thousands of health professionals strike over manpower shortage (*The Times of Israel*, 27 May 2018)

12. Reis et al., Medical education in Israel 2016: five medical schools in a period of transition, *Israel Journal of Health Policy Research*, 5(45) (2016)

13. Siegel-Itzkovich J, University of Haifa program lets degree-holders become nurses in less time (*The Jerusalem Post*, 12 September 2017)

14. State of Israel Ministry of Health, Physician Assistants (2018)

15. Berkowitz O, Jacobson E, Fire G, & Afek A, Physician assistants in Israel, *Journal of the American Academy of Physician Assistants*, 27(12), 7–8 (2014)

16. Ministry of Health announces healthcare startup pilot program in Israel (Dr. Hempel Digital Health Network, 27 June 2018)

17. Clalit Health Services, Online pediatrician

18. Waisman Y, Telemedicine in pediatric emergency care: an overview and description of a novel service in Israel, *Journal of Intensive and Critical Care*, 2(2) (2016)

19. Eilat-Tsanani et al., Evaluation of telehealth service for patients with congestive heart failure in the north of Israel, *European Journal of Cardiovascular Nursing*, 15(3), 78–84 (2016)

20. TytoCare Partners with Israel's Clalit Health Service Organization, No Camels News, 25 February 2018

Chapter 5

1. Desjardins, J, The US spends more public money on healthcare than Sweden or Canada (*Visual Capitalist*, 31 March 2017)

2. OECD, Health workforce policies in OECD countries, Right jobs, right skills, right places (2016)

3. KPMG International, Value walks: successful habits for improving workforce motivation and productivity in healthcare, 2016

4. Kentish B, How reliant is the NHS on foreign doctors? (*Independent*, 4 June 2018)

5. UCAS data, 23 October 2017

6. Press Association, NHS cap on trainee doctors should be scrapped, think tank says (*Daily Mail*, 14 September 2017)

7. Double or quits: calculating how many more medical students we need (Royal College of Physicians, June 2018)

8. OECD, Health workforce policies in OECD countries, Australia (March 2016)

9. Weinbren E, England faces surplus of 19,000 pharmacists by 2040 (*Chemist and Druggist*, 5 September 2013)

10. The Health Foundation, Fit for purpose? Workforce policy in the English NHS (The Health Foundation, 2016)

11. Department of Health and Social Care, Promoting professionalism, reforming regulation: a paper for consultation (UK Department of Health and Social Care, 2017)

12. Rauhala E, Why China's doctors are getting beat up (*Time*, 7 March 2014)

13. GBD 2016 SDG Collaborators, Measuring progress and projecting attainment on the basis of past trends of the health-related Sustainable Development Goals in 188 countries: an analysis from the Global Burden of Disease Study 2016, *The Lancet*, 390(10100), 1423–59 (2017)

14. WHO and World Economic Forum, From burden to 'best buys': reducing the economic impact of noncommunicable diseases in low- and middle-income countries (World Economic Forum, 2011)

15. WHO, Health employment and economic growth: an evidence base, Chapter 11, p. 266

16. Health workforce policies in OECD countries: right jobs, right skills, right places, OECD Health Policy Studies (OECD, 2016)

Chapter 6

1. Economist Intelligence Unit, Healthcare report: China (EIU, 2017)

2. World Industry Outlook: Healthcare, Economist Intelligence Unit, 4th Quarter 2018

3. Jie H, Chinese hospitals aiming to recruit more male nurses despite stigma (*CGTN*, 12 May 2017)

4. Xinhua, 20 August 2018

5. Yue Z, General practitioner plan set to meet rising demand in China (*China Daily*, 23 May 2017)

6. Stanway D, China to boost beds, staff to handle healthcare strains (*Reuters*, 11 January 2017)

7. Xiaodong W, Children paying price for shortage of doctors (*China Daily*, 3 March 2017)

8. Wu et al., Shortage of healthcare professionals in China, *British Medical Journal*, 354, i4860 (September 2016)

9. Liu Y, Chinese doctor stabbed to death after row with patient's husband (*South China Morning Post*, 15 March 2018)

10. Li J, China's private hospitals struggle to attract top physicians (*South China Morning Post*, 27 March 2017)

11. KPMG, Sanming: the real story of grass-roots healthcare transformation in China, 28 November 2016

12. Jourdan A, AI ambulances and robot doctors: China seeks digital salve to ease hospital strain (*Reuters*, 28 June 2018)

13. Li J & Benitez MA, Tencent-backed health care platform WeDoctor shrugs off bear market concerns, prepares for Hong Kong IPO (*South China Morning Post*, 10 July 2018)

14. Zhu J, Ping An's Good Doctor unit raises $1.1 billion in Hong Kong IPO: sources (*Reuters*, 27 April 2018)

15. Sun Y, AI could alleviate China's doctor shortage (*MIT Technology Review*, 21 March 2018)

16. Huang E, This Chinese hospital is putting its patients in the hands of AI (World Economic Forum, 6 April 2018)

17. Jourdan A, AI ambulances and robot doctors: China seeks digital salve to ease hospital strain (*Reuters*, 28 June 2018)

18. Lifang, China's AI-general practitioner system starts hospital trial (*Xinhua Net*, 5 March 2018)

19. Sun Y, AI could alleviate China's doctor shortage (*MIT Technology Review*, 21 March 2018)

Chapter 7

1. Morioka et al., The business case for people powered health (Nesta, 2013)

2. Pruitt S & Jordan E, Preparing the 21st century global healthcare workforce, *British Medical Journal*, 330, 637 (2005)

3. The Institute for Public Policy Research, Powerful people: Reinforcing the power of citizens and communities in health and care (IPPR, 2015)

4. Hampson M, Redefining consultations: changing the relationships at the heart of health (Nesta, 2013)

5. Ibid.

6. Rogers et al., National evaluation of the pilot phase of the expert patients programme final report (National Primary Care Research & Development Centre, 2006)

7. Durcan et al., The future of the mental health workforce (NHS Confederation Mental Health Network, 2017)

8. NHS Confederation, Reducing hospital admissions among high users of urgent care (NHS Vale of York Clinical Commissioning Group, 2017)

9. 5 Benefits of self-service kiosks in hospitals (Techadvisory.org, 1 April 2016)

10. Imperial College Health Partners, Diabetes Digital Behavior Change Programmes: North West London Pilot (2018)

11. Vize R, Unleashing the power of digital patient (Digital Health London, 25 April 2017)

12. Organization for Economic Cooperation and Development, The impact of caring on family carers (OECD, 2011)

13. Ibid.

14. Gottlieb K, The Nuka system of care: improving health through ownership and relationships, *International Journal of Circumpolar Health*, 5, 72 (2013)

15. Prost et al., Women's groups practising participatory learning and action to improve maternal and new-born health in low-resource settings: a systematic review and meta-analysis, *Lancet*, 381(9879), 1736–46, (2013)

Chapter 8

1. OECD statistics, Long term care expenditure in Health at a Glance 2017 (OECD, 2017)

2. OECD statistics, The Netherlands—a good life in old age (OECD, 2013)

3. Kroneman M, Boerma W, van den Berg M, Groenewegen P, de Jong J, & van Ginneken E, The Netherlands: health system review, *Health Systems in Transition*, 18(2) (2016)

4. PwC, Dutch Innovation Survey 2017 (PWC, 2017)

5. Kroneman et al., 2016.

6. Arie S, Why are Dutch GPs so much happier? (*British Medical Journal*, 2015)

7. Ibid.

8. The Commonwealth Fund, Home care by self-governing nursing teams: the Netherlands' Buurtzorg Model (2015)

9. Kroneman et al., 2016

10. Nederlands instituut voor onderzoek van de gezondheidszorg, Health workforce planning in Netherlands (NIVEL, 2016)

11. Ibid.

12. Batenburg R, The Dutch model of health human resources planning and the new challenges of an integrative European perspective, *European Journal of Public Health*, 23 (2013)

13. Ibid.

14. Kroneman et al., 2016

15. Europe—Demand for nursing staff on the rise, UK sees biggest shortage of nurses (Staffing Industry Analysts, 12 January 2018)

Chapter 9

1. Desjardins J, Germany will hit a significant demographic milestone over the next year (World Economic Forum, 18 January 2018)

2. World Health Organization, Current health expenditure, WHO Global Health Expenditure Database (2000–2015)

3. OECD statistics, Doctors and nurses per 1,000 population (OECD, 2016)

4. Dussault et al., Assessing future health workforce needs (WHO, 2010)

5. Health policy overview: health policy in Germany (OECD, July 2016)

6. OECD indicators, Health at a Glance 2015, Hip and knee replacements (Chapter 6) (OECD, 2015)

7. European Observatory on Health Systems and Policies, State of Health in the EU—Germany (OECD, 2017)

8. Kopetsch T, The migration of doctors to and from Germany, *Journal of Public Health*, 17(1) (February 2009)

9. European Observatory on Health Systems and Policies, Health systems in transition profile of Germany

10. OECD International Migration Outlook, 2015

11. Knight B, German home care rules leave gaps for off-the-books work (*Deutsche Welle*, 8 August 2018)

12. Ibid.

13. World Health Organization Regional Office for Europe, The toolkit for a sustainable health workforce in the WHO European region, 2018

14. GIZ—[Deutsche gesellschaft für internationale zusammenarbeit], Training nurses from Viet Nam to become geriatric nurses in Germany (GIZ, 2016)

15. Brady K, Who will look after us? (DW.com, 16 July 2018)

16. Rhee et al., Considering long-term care insurance for middle-income countries: comparing South Korea with Japan and Germany, *Health Policy*, 119(10), 1319–29 (October 2015)

17. Centre for Policy on Ageing, International case study 8: long-term care insurance in Germany (January 2016)

18. Lutz & Palenga-Möllenbeck, *Care Work Migration in Germany: Semi Compliance and Complicity* (*Cambridge University Press*, 2010)

19. *Deutsche Welle*, Germany to recruit more elderly care workers abroad (*Deutsche Welle*, 31 March 2018)

20. The long-term care workforce: overview and strategies to adapt supply to a growing demand (OECD, 2009)

21. Kuhlmann et al., Regional health workforce monitoring as governance innovation: a German model to coordinate sectoral demand, skill mix and mobility, *Human Resources for Health*, 14, 71 (2016)

Chapter 10

1. Health workforce policies in OECD countries: right jobs, right skills, right places (OECD, 2016)

2. Programme for the International Assessment of Adult Competencies (OECD, 2012)

3. Nurses swamped by paperwork (*Telegraph*, 21 April 2013)

4. Eastman T, PACK—the Practical Approach to Care Kit, BMJ Clinical Evidence (*British Medical Journal*, 14 January 2016)

5. Sharma S, Oncologist, entrepreneur, startup mentor: how HCG's Dr Ajaikumar is using technology to transform cancer care (*Your Story*, 11 June 2018)

6. Driving down the cost of high-quality care: lessons from the Aravind Eye Care System (McKinsey, 2011)

7. Wright et al., Beyond burnout — redesigning care to restore meaning and sanity for physicians, *The New England Journal of Medicine*, 378, 309–11 (January, 2015)

8. OECD, Health Workforce Policies in OECD countries (OECD, 2016)

9. Imison C, Castle-Clarke S, & Watson R, Reshaping the workforce to deliver the care patients need. Research Report (Nuffield Trust, 2016)

10. New medicine course in West Cumbria is 'first of its kind' in the UK (*Cumbria Crack*, 6 January 2018)

11. Dubois & Singh, From staff-mix to skill-mix and beyond: towards a systemic approach to health workforce management, US National Library of Medicine (National Institute of Health, 2009)

12. OECD, Health Workforce Policies in OECD countries (OECD, 2016)

13. Abbott A, *The System of Professions* (University of Chicago Press, 2014)

14. Krause E, *Death of Gilds* (Yale University Press, 1999)

15. Aiken et al., Nursing skill mix in European hospitals: cross-sectional study of the association with mortality, patient ratings, and quality of care, *BMJ Journals* (2016)

16. Gray B, Home care by self-governing nursing teams: the Netherlands' Buurtzorg model, The Commonwealth Fund (29 May 2015)

17. UNICEF, The number of newborns worldwide dying in the first month of life is 3.3 million (UNICEF, 2010)

18. Lund et al., Mobile phone intervention reduces perinatal mortality in Zanzibar: secondary outcomes of a cluster randomized controlled trial, JMIR mHealth and uHealth (2014)

19. Rogan F, What can the assembly line teach us about innovation? (*Raidió Teilifís Éireann RTE*, 12 March 2018)

20. General Medical Council consultation on credentialing, 2015

21. The Health Foundation, A year of plenty? An analysis of NHS finances and consultant productivity (NHS, 2016)

22. Ibid.

23. Lyon et al., A team-based care model that improves job satisfaction (American Academy of Family Physicians, March 2018)

24. Thouin MF & Bardhan I, The effect of information systems on the quality and cost of healthcare processes: a longitudinal study of U.S. hospitals. In: ICIS Proceedings, 2009 Paper 64

25. Tursunbayeva et al., Human resource information systems in health care: a systematic evidence review, *Journal of the American Medical Informatics Association*, 24(3), 633–54 (1 May 2017)

26. World Health Organization, More health for the money (Chapter 4) (WHO, 2010)

Chapter 11

1. McConnell, Staff turnover: occasional friend, frequent foe, and continuing frustration, *Europe PMC*, 18(1), 1–13 (1999)

2. Lo et al., A systematic review of burnout among doctors in China: a cultural perspective, *Asia Pacific Family Medicine*, 17(3) (2018)

3. Holland P & Tham T-L, Burnt-out and overworked, Australia's nurses and midwives consider leaving profession (*The Conversation*, 28 September 2016)

4. Aiken et al., Patient safety, satisfaction, and quality of hospital care: cross sectional surveys of nurses and patients in 12 countries in Europe and the United States, *British Medical Journal* (2012)

5. Deloitte Centre for Health Solutions, Time to care: securing a future for the hospital workforce in Europe (Deloitte, 2017)

6. More UK nurses and midwives leaving than joining profession, BBC News (3 July 2017)

7. Wu et al., Health system reforms, violence against doctors and job satisfaction in the medical profession: a cross-sectional survey in Zhejiang Province, Eastern China, *BMJ Journals* (2014)

8. Irving et al., International variations in primary care physician consultation time: a systematic review of 67 countries, *BMJ Journals* (2017)

9. 2016 Survey of America's Physicians: Practice Patterns & Perspectives (The Physicians Foundation, 2016)

10. Lakshman S, Nurse turnover in India: factors impacting nurses' decisions to leave employment, *South Asian Journal of Human Resources Management* (November, 2016)

11. Yang et al., Validation of work pressure and associated factors influencing hospital nurse turnover: a cross-sectional investigation in Shaanxi Province, China, US National Library of Medicines (National Institutes of Health, 2017)

12. Tamil Nadu government doctors to go on one day strike on May 8 (*New Indian Express*, 1 May 2017)

13. Facing the Facts, Shaping the Future, Health Education England (NHS, 2017)

14. Price Waterhouse Coopers, PWC's NextGen: a global generational study (PWC, 2013)

15. Park SH, Gass S, & Boyle DK, Comparison of reasons for nurse turnover in Magnet® and non-Magnet hospitals, *The Journal of Nursing Administration*, 46(5), 284–90 (2016)

16. McHugh MD, Wage, work environment and staffing: effects on nurse outcomes, *US National Library of Medicines* (National Institutes of Health, 2013)

17. Hayes et al., Nurse turnover: a literature review, *International Journal of Nursing Studies*, 43(2) (2006)

18. Twigg & Kylie, Nurse retention: a review of strategies to create and enhance positive practice environments in clinical settings, *International Journal of Nursing Studies*, 51(1) (2014)

19. Feeley D, Joy in work: more than the absence of burnout, Institute for Healthcare Improvement, Institute for Healthcare Improvement (1 August 2017)

20. NHS Employers, Improving staff retention: a guide for employers (NHS, 2017)

21. Frimley Health, NHS Foundation Trust, Annual Report and Accounts (NHS, 2016–2017)

22. Deloitte, Continuous performance management (Deloitte, 2017)

23. Improving the NHS with the Getting it Right First Time Programme (DAC Beachcroft, 20 October 2017)

24. Jee C, New Cross Hospital installs location tracking technology (*Computer World UK*, 1 July 2014)

25. Blair M, Nearly one in five new nurses leaves first job within a year, according to survey of newly-licensed registered nurses (RobertWood Johnson Foundation, 4 September 2017)

26. CapitalNurse reflecting—How do you value preceptorship? (NHS, 2017)

27. Royal College of Nursing, Investing in a Safe and Effective Workforce (RCN, 2018)

28. Find great places to work—top-rated workplaces (Indeed.com, 2018)

29. National Council of State Boards of Nursing, National nursing workforce study 2015

30. Golbuff L & Aldred R, Cycling policy in the UK—a historical and thematic overview, *UEL Sustainable Mobilities Research Group* (2011)

31. RAND Corporation, Providing support to the Britain's healthiest workplace competition (2015)

32. Business Action on Health, Healthy people = healthy profits (Business in the Community, 2016)

33. Chartered Institute of Personnel and Development (CIPD), CIPD submission to the Independent Review (CIPD, 2016)

34. Avantas client stories: the University of Kansas Hospital (16 August 2017)

Chapter 12

1. World Health Organization, Working for health and growth (WHO, 2016)

2. Real Man's Work, Male Nurses Worldwide (5 May 2012)

3. OECD, Health statistics (OECD, 2016)

4. Ramakrishnan et al., Women's participation in the medical profession: insights from experiences in Japan, Scandinavia, Russia, and Eastern Europe, *Journal of Women's Health*, 23(11) (2014)

5. OECD, 2016

6. Ramakrishnan et al., 2014

7. Levy H, How the gender gap is shifting in medicine, by specialty (Amino, 14 September 2018)

8. Bedoya-Vaca et al., Gender and physician specialization and practice settings in Ecuador: a qualitative study, *BMC Health Services Research* (2016)

9. Peckham C, Medscape female physician compensation report, Medscape (17 May 2017)

10. Ly DP, Seabury SA, & Jena AB, Hours worked among US dual physician couples with children, 2000 to 2015, *JAMA International Medicine*, 177(10), 1524–5 (2017)

11. General Medical Council, What our data tells us about general practitioners working for the NHS in England and Scotland (GMC, May 2018)

12. Baird et al., Understanding pressures in General Practice, King's Fund (The King's Fund, 5 May 2016)

13. Donnelly L, GP shortage fuelled by rising numbers working part-time, *Telegraph* (15 June 2017)

14. Van Hassel et al., Age-related differences in working hours among male and female GPs: an SMS-based time use study, *Human Resources for Health*, 15(1), 84 (2017)

15. Lautenberger et al., The state of women in academic medicine, Association of American Medical Colleges (2014)

16. Wehner et al., Plenty of moustaches but not enough women: cross sectional study of medical leaders, *British Medical Journal*, 351 (2015)

17. Cavallo J, Overcoming sexism in academic medicine, *The ASCO Post* (10 July 2017)

18. Ramakrishnan et al., 2014

19. Kavilanz P, The gender pay gap for women doctors is big— and getting worse, *CNN Money* (14 March 2018)

20. Triggle N, Top women doctors lose out in NHS pay stakes, *BBC* (16 February 2018)

21. Kaneto et al., Gender difference in physician workforce participation in Japan, *Health Policy*, 89(1), 115–23 (2008)

22. The World Bank, Women, business, and the law 2016: getting to equal (World Bank, 2016)

23. Kates et al., Health and access to care and coverage for lesbian, gay, bisexual and transgender individuals in the US, The Henry J. Kaiser Family Foundation (2015)

24. Childcare costs: survey by Mumsnet and the Resolution Foundation, Mumsnet, 2017

25. Rudner LN, Full practice authority for advanced practice registered nurses is a gender issue, *Online Journal of Issues in Nursing*, 21(2), 6 (2016)

26. Miller CC, Pink-collar jobs: why men don't want the jobs done mostly by women, *The Sydney Morning Herald*, 6 January 2017

Chapter 13

1. OECD Statistics, Better Life Index (OECD, 2017)

2. Smith J, Australia curbs flow of disgruntled UK junior doctors (*Financial Times*, 1 November 2016)

3. Sabin S, 10 highest paid countries in the world for doctors, Medic footprints (28 July 2016)

4. Australian Medical Association, Managing the risk of fatigue in the medical workforce (AMA, 2016)

5. Phoraris S, Top 10 countries with the highest paid salaries for nurses (*Career Addict*, 2 January 2017)

6. Rural Australia missing out on doctors—AMA calls on government to lift training targets (Australian Medical Association, 3 December 2015)

7. Australian Medical Association, Regional inequality in Australia (Submission 77) (AMA, 2018)

8. Australian Govt. Department of Health, Rural Junior Doctor Training Innovation Fund (MoH, 4 January 2018)

9. Australian Govt. Department of Health, General Practice Rural Incentives Program (GPRIP) (MoH, 24 April 2018)

10. Queensland Government, Queensland Rural Generalist Pathway: what it was, is and must become (2018)

11. The Council of Australian Governments Health Council, Independent review of accreditation systems within the National Registration and Accreditation Scheme for health professions (COAG, 2017)

12. Parnell S, Medical training reforms and getting doctors in the regions (*The Australian*, 4 November 2017)

13. Victoria's Hub for health services and business, Advanced practice programs (Department of Health & Human Services, 2017)

14. Australian Institute of Health and Welfare, Mental Health Services in Australia (AIHW, July 2018)

15. Crettenden et al., How evidence-based workforce planning in Australia is informing policy development in the retention and distribution of the health workforce, *Human Resources for Health* (2014)

16. Australian Institute for Health and Welfare, Mortality and life expectancy of Indigenous Australians 2008 to 2012 (AIHW, 2014)

17. Achieving Aboriginal and Torres Strait Islander health equality within a generation—a human rights-based approach, Australian Human Rights Association (2005)

18. Bradford N, Caffery L, & Smith A, Telehealth services in rural and remote Australia: a systematic review of models of care and factors influencing success and sustainability, *Rural and Remote Health*, 16, 3808 (2016)

19. Bindi T, How Australia can overcome multiple barriers to drive telehealth adoption (ZDNet, 5 April 2017)

Chapter 14

1. Charlesworth A & Johnson P, Securing the future: funding health and social care to the 2030, Institute for Fiscal Studies, NHS Confederation (May 2018)

2. Ibid.

3. Ham C & Murray R, The NHS 10-year plan: how should the extra funding be spent? (The King's Fund, 12 July 2018)

4. Campbell D, NHS suffering worst ever staff and cash crisis, figures show (*The Guardian*, 11 September 2018)

5. Helm T, May to unveil £20bn a year boost to NHS spending (*The Observer*, 16 June 2018)

6. The general practice forward view: two years on (British Medical Association, 2018)

7. Facing the Facts, Shaping the Future, A draft health and care workforce strategy for England to 2027 (Health Education England, 2017)

Chapter 15

1. De Fauw et al., Clinically applicable deep learning for diagnosis and referral in the retinal disease, *Nature Medicine* (2018)

2. Boston Consulting Group (BCG), Reshaping business with artificial intelligence (2017)

3. McKinsey & Company, A future that works: automation, employment, and productivity (2017)

4. Himmelstein et al., A comparison of hospital administrative costs in eight nations (Commonwealth Fund, September 2014)

5. Thanks to my KPMG colleague Robert Bolton for his insights on AI, set out in evidence to the UK All Party Parliamentary Group on artificial intelligence, 26 February 2018

6. Spears M, Bolton R, & Brown D, Rise of the humans 2 (KPMG, 2017)

7. Goodwin B, Employers face hiring crisis as AI replaces mid-skilled jobs (*Computer Weekly*, 16 March 2018)

8. Calme G, Artificial intelligence in clinical decision-making: will it cure the field of medicine? (ResearchGate, April 2016)

9. Vize R, Healthtech: the opportunities and the risks (*Digital Health London*, 3 March 2017)

10. Billington J, IBM's Watson cracks medical mystery with life-saving diagnosis for patient who baffled doctors (*International Business Times*, 8 August 2018)

11. Herper M, MD Anderson benches IBM Watson in setback for Artificial Intelligence in medicine (*Forbes*, 19 February 2017)

12. Calme, 2016

13. Sennaar K, How America's 5 top hospitals are using machine learning today (techemergence.com, 13 April 2018)

14. Tempus and Mayo Clinic team up to personalize care for cancer patients (CISION PR Newswire, 4 January 2017)

15. Cleveland Clinic to identify at-risk patients in ICU using Cortana intelligence (*ML Blog Team*, 26 September 2016)

16. NVIDIA, Massachusetts General Hospital use AI to advance radiology, pathology, genomics (*HPCwire*, 5 April 2016)

17. Willcocks et al., *The IT Function and Robotic Process Automation* (The Outsourcing Unit, LSE, 2015)

18. Bean R, Will blockchain transform healthcare (*Forbes*, 5 August 2018)

Chapter 16

1. Masutomo T, Japan's open to foreign workers. Just don't call them immigrants (*SCMP*, 30 June 2018); see also OECD, Japan: promoting inclusive growth for an ageing society, Better Policy Series (OECD, April 2018)

2. Gros D, Centre for European Policy Studies, Demographic lessons from Japan for Europe (CEPS, November 2017)

3. World Bank statistics, Age Dependency Ratio (World Bank, 2017)

4. International Monetary Fund, Japan: at a glance (International Monetary Fund, 2018)

5. OECD statistics, Doctors per 1,000 inhabitants (OECD, 2017)

6. OECD statistics, Nurses per 1,000 inhabitants (OECD, 2017)

7. Shortage of nursing care workers (*The Japan Times*, 7 July 2015)

8. Henke et al., Improving Japan's health care system, McKinsey (March, 2009)

9. Ibid.

10. Japan's robot industry for elderly encouraged by Government (*The Tokyo Times*, 2013)

11. Japan is ill prepared for coming labour shock (*The Financial Times*, 9 January 2018)

12. World Health Organization, Japan Health System Review, Health Systems in Transition, Vol. 8 No 1 (WHO, 2018)

13. OECD Reviews of Health Care Quality: Japan 2015 (OECD, 2015)

14. OECD statistics, Length of hospital stay (OECD, 2017)

15. OECD statistics, Doctor's consultations (OECD, 2017)

16. OECD statistics, Hospital beds (OECD, 2017)

Chapter 17

1. Daly M, Obama is not the first President to fight the health care fight (*New York Daily News*, 10 September 2009)

2. OECD, Coverage for health care—Health at a glance 2015: OECD Indicators (OECD, 2015)

3. National Rural Health Association, About rural health care (NRHA, 2016)

4. Topol EJ & Emanuel E, No physician shortage despite dire warnings: Zeke Emanuel (*Medscape*, 24 January 2018)

5. OECD statistics, Physicians by categories: density per 1,000 population (OECD, 2016)

6. Medscape's 2018 Physician Compensation Report

7. Association of American Medical Colleges, 2018 education debt manager: for graduating medical school students (AAMC, 2018)

8. Health Resources and Services Administration, Projecting the supply and demand for primary care practitioners through 2020 (HRSA, 2013)

9. FutureDocs Forecasting Tool & Cecil G. Sheps Center for Health Services Research, University of North Carolina

10. Where the states stand on Medicaid expansion (Advisory Board, 8 June 2018)

11. Center for Healthcare Research and Transformation, Affordable Care Act Funding: an analysis of grant programs under health care reform (CHRT, 2012)

12. Biviano MB, Tise S, & Dall TM, What is behind HRSA's projected U.S. supply, demand, and shortages of registered nurses, *Modelling Our Future: Population Ageing, Health and Aged Care, 2007*, 343–374 (2007)

13. Ibid.

14. Goodman DC, Twenty-year trends in regional variations in the U.S. physician workforce, *Health Affairs* VAR90-VAR97 (2004)

15. Papanicolas I, Woskie LR, & Jha AK, Health care spending in the United States and other high-income countries, *Journal of the American Medical Association*, 319(10), 1024–39 (2018)

16. Ibid.

17. National Health Expenditure Data: Historical, US Centers for Medicare & Medicaid Services, 8 January 2018

18. Congress of the United States Congressional Budget Office, Federal Subsidies for Health Insurance Coverage for People Under Age 65: 2018 to 2028 (CBO, 2018)

19. Mercer M, Is your Medicare safe? (AARP Bulletin, January 2014)

20. Papanicolas I, Woskie LR, & Jha AK, Health care spending in the United States and other high-income countries, *Journal of the American Medical Association*, 319(10), 1024–39 (2018)

21. Diamond D, Ready to get your drugs by drone? Why Amazon plan could be game-changer (*Forbes*, 20 March 2015)

22. A merger between CVS Health and Aetna could be what the doctor ordered (*The Economist*, 4 November 2017)

Chapter 18

1. World Health Organization, Factsheets: Universal Health Coverage (UHC) (WHO, 2017)

2. World Innovation Summit for Health, Delivering Universal Health Coverage: a guide for policymakers (WISH, 2015)

3. Pasma J, Ten years of *Seguro Popular* (*Salud Mexico*, 2 September 2014)

4. Gustavo et al., Evaluating the implementation of Mexico's health reform: the case of Seguro Popular, *Health Systems and Reforms*, 1(3), 217–8 (2015)

5. Urquieta-Salomón JE & Héctor JV, Evolution of health coverage in Mexico: evidence of progress and challenges in the Mexican health system, *Journal of Health Policy and Planning* (2015)

6. World Health Organization, Thailand—Country cooperation strategy: at a glance (WHO, 2010)

7. Khan JF, Romanians despair that wealthy Britain is taking all their doctors (*Financial Times*, 14 January 2014)

8. Romanian Govt. to increase doctors' salaries by over 70% (*Romanian Insider*, 9 February 2018)

9. Ibid.

10. Alexe A, Higher salaries starting today for some public sector workers (*Business Review*, 1 March 2018)

11. Assefa et al., Health system's response for physician workforce shortages and the upcoming crisis in Ethiopia: a grounded theory research, *Human Resources for Health* (BMC, 2017)

12. World Health Organization, Health Heroes + Social Good Summit (WHO, 2018)

13. World Bank, Tracking universal health coverage: 2017 global monitoring report (World Bank, 2017)

14. Applying technology and innovation to produce world class physicians cost effectively delivering superior health outcomes (Global Medical University, 2017)

15. Shetty D & Kumar V, A global university can be a shot in the arm for medical teaching (*Hindustan Times*, 8 April 2016)

16. Moon R & Shin G-W, From brain drain to brain circulation and linkage (Freeman Spogli Institute of International Studies, 2018)

17. The Wharton School: management, How Cuba's Health Care Sector aims to gain a greater foothold (in collaboration with Transactional Track Record, 2015)

18. Alves L, Brazil's Mais medicos program to lose Cuban Doctors (*The Rio Times*, 4 October 2017)

19. The Philippines' health worker exodus (*The Lancet*, 2009)

20. Hapal DK, Why our nurses are leaving (*Rappler*, 2 September 2017)

21. Cheng MH, The Philippines' health worker exodus, *The Lancet*, world report, 373(9658) (10 January 2009)

22. Sood et al., Causes, consequences, and policy responses to the migration of health workers: key findings from India, *Human Resources for Health* (2017)

23. Kohlway E, Stemming the tide of African health worker migration (Global Health Council, 13 December 2011)

24. Department for International Development, UK announces major investments in future of African youth through education and voluntary family planning (Gov.UK, 2018)

25. Kigotho W, African Union devises 10 year plan to stem brain drain (*University World News*, 9 February 2018)

26. We have made medical education elitist, out of reach of poor families. It will have consequences: Cardiac Surgeon Devi Shetty (*The Indian Express*, 24 December 2017)

27. Imperial College of London, Evaluating the impact of private providers on health and health systems (Global Health Innovation, 2017)

28. Non-state actors in higher education in Sri Lanka: issues and challenges (*Daily Mirror*, 27 February 2017)

29. Weerasinghe C, UK Medical Council says SAITM qualification unacceptable (*Daily News*, 15 September 2017)

30. SAITM abolished (*Daily Mirror*, 29 October 2017)

31. KPMG, What works: the triple win—rethinking public private partnerships for universal healthcare (KPMG, 2017)

32. Russell J, Telecom giant Telenor launches a digital health service for emerging markets (*Tech Crunch*, 2016)

Chapter 19

1. World Health Organization, Brazil: country cooperation strategy (WHO, May 2018)

2. Buchan J, Fronteira I, & Dussault G, Continuity and change in human resources policies for health: lessons from Brazil, *Human Resources for Health*, 9(17) (2011)

3. Ibid.

4. World Health Organization, Density of physicians (WHO, 2018)

5. Ibid.

6. Scheffer MC & Dal Poz MR, The privatization of medical education in Brazil: trends and challenges, *Human Resources for Health*, 13(96) (2015)

7. Buchan J, Fronteira I, & Dussault G, Continuity and change in human resources policies for health: lessons from Brazil, *Human Resources for Health*, 9(17) (2011)

8. Community workers are the key to improved health in Brazil, University of York (11 April 2017)

9. WHO country cooperation strategy, Brazil

10. Wadge H, Brazil's Family Health Strategy: using community healthcare workers to provide primary care (The Commonwealth Fund, 13 December 2016)

11. National Association of Private Hospitals (ANAHP), Medical Demography Research in Brazil, 2015

12. Ibid.

13. Bevins V, Brazil's president imports Cuban doctors to ease shortage (*Los Angeles Times*, 6 January 2014)

14. Buchan et al., Continuity and change in human resources policies for health: lessons from Brazil, *Human Resources for Health*, 9, 17 (2011)

15. Chieffi AL, Barradas RDCB, & Golbaum M, Legal access to medications: a threat to Brazil's public health system?, *BMC Health Services Research*, 17(1), 499 (2017)

16. Massuda A, The Brazilian health system at crossroads: progress, crisis and resilience, *BMJ Global Health*, 5 June 2018

17. Cardoso et al., Understanding Brazil's workforce in a troubled time, *BCG*, 17 March 2016

18. Gragnolati M, Twenty years of health system reform in Brazil, an assessment of the Sistema Único de Saúde, The World Bank (2013)

19. Ibid.

20. What the US can learn from Brazil's healthcare mess (*The Atlantic*, 8 May 2014)

21. Stripoli G, LATAM to reach 2.5bn mobile devices by 2025; Mexican digital ad market grows by 28% (*Exchange Wire*, 4 September 2017)

22. Collucci C, Brazil's child and maternal mortality have increased against background of public spending cuts, *British Medical Journal*, 362, k3583 (2018)

Chapter 20

1. OECD statistics, Historical population data and projections: elderly population (OECD, 2015)
2. Statistics Norway, Employed persons 15–74 years: by sex and industry division (Statistics Norway, 2017)
3. Hellenic Statistical Authority statistics, Labor force survey yearly time series: by sector (Hellenic Statistical Authority, 2017)
4. OECD statistics, Labor force participation rate: by sex (OECD, 2017)
5. KPMG, What works: creating new value with patients, carers and communities (KPMG, 2014)
6. Nesta, The business case for people powered health (Nesta, 2013)
7. Institute and Faculty of Actuaries, Long-term care reform in Germany—at long last (Institute and Faculty of Actuaries, 2017)
8. Ibid.
9. World Health Organization, Health employment and economic growth: an evidence base (WHO, 2017)
10. National Health Service, Working in the NHS (NHS, 2018)
11. Forrester Research, The future of jobs, 2025: working side by side with robots (Forrester, 2015)
12. Topol E, Preparing the healthcare workforce to deliver the digital future: Interim Report June 2018—a call for evidence, *National Health Service* (2018)
13. McKinsey Global Institute, Jobs lost, jobs gained: workforce transitions in a time of automation (McKinsey, 2017)
14. National Health Services Digital statistics, Healthcare Workforce Statistics (NHS, 2018)
15. West M, Both staff and patients need care, compassion and respect (*Nursing Times*, 8 January 2014)

Index